Intermittent Fasting for Women Over 50

The Ultimate Step-by-Step Guide for Beginners.
Lose Weight Effectively, Boost Your Energy,
and Turn Back The Clock.

Recipes and Meal Plan Included

Emily Walker

Contents

Introduction

Aging is an unavoidable part of life. As you age, you go through different physiological changes ranging from reduction in energy levels to hormonal changes. That said, the one constant is your responsibility to your health. Your well-being lies in your hands. Consuming a healthy and wholesome diet, exercising regularly, getting sufficient sleep at night, and managing stress levels are crucial for leading a healthy and happy life.

Women experiencing menopause and those close to or who have reached the big five-oh will experience different changes. Most of them are associated with a shift in the basic hormonal composition and makeup. The good news is these changes don't have to hold you back or prevent you from leading your life to the fullest. Once you reach and cross the big five-oh, your life changes in more ways than ever expected; maybe you are trying to reassert your independence now that your kids are away. Perhaps you are going

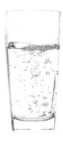

through menopause and trying to make the most of the few years left before retirement. Maybe you are worried about retaining your well-groomed image while experiencing menopause-related physical changes. If you gained a few extra pounds around the abdominal region and are worried about it, then you are not alone. During and after menopause, a common complaint most women have is belly fat. It can be quite disconcerting to see yourself out of shape, which is a source of added stress.

Going through menopause might not sound like much; however, all the physiological changes accompanying it will change your life. From weight gain to mood swings and hot flashes are all associated with the changes in hormonal composition your body is experiencing. Well, the only thing you need to do is start taking care of your health by concentrating on your diet. Selecting the right diet is not easy these days, given the number of options available. Most conventional diets prescribe several calorie restrictions; they are restrictive and seldom sustainable. A combination of these factors makes it difficult to follow the diet. Even if you do, the results aren't sustainable once you stop following the dietary protocols. But you don't have to worry because you are not alone. Life can be stressful at times, but your diet doesn't have to be.

During menopause, you may have realized that you are no longer as active as you once used to be. Keeping yourself healthy and fit is not as simple as it was during your twenties. Changing your dietary patt

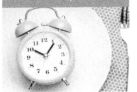

erns and following a conventional diet is not easy and seems downright impossible. All this merely increases the stress you are already experiencing. On your quest to find the right diet, you might have stumbled across several unsustainable ones. You probably want to lose those pesky extra pounds that are preventing you from feeling good about yourself. You want to feel good about yourself and feel attractive again but are struggling to find the starting point. Well, you are not alone! Are you wondering how I know all this? Well, I believe a little introduction is needed. Hello, my name is Emily Walker. I am a happily married woman in my fifties with a wonderful family. Going through menopause taught me a lot about my body and myself in general. I didn't want my life to be guided by physiological changes beyond my control. Instead, I decided to take charge of my health by concentrating on simple dietary changes. This was when I discovered the power of intermittent fasting.

Intermittent fasting is a simple dietary protocol that oscillates between eating and fasting. In this book, you will learn about the concept of intermittent fasting, its different variations, popular myths about it, and all the different benefits it offers. As you age, different physiological changes start taking place within your body. These changes not only reflect physically but change the internal mechanisms too.

You will learn about simple suggestions that can be used while fasting, after fasting, and tips to break a fast.

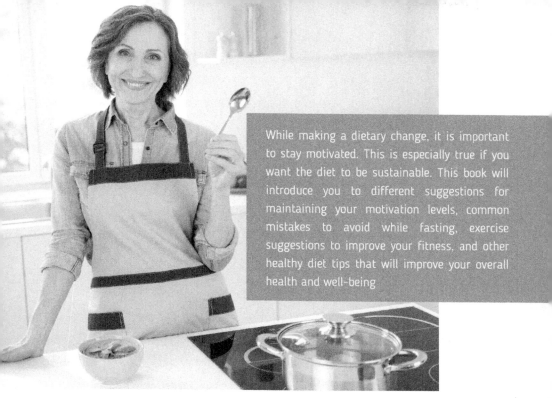

While making a dietary change, it is important to stay motivated. This is especially true if you want the diet to be sustainable. This book will introduce you to different suggestions for maintaining your motivation levels, common mistakes to avoid while fasting, exercise suggestions to improve your fitness, and other healthy diet tips that will improve your overall health and well-being

You will discover several intermittent fasting friendly meal options in this book. All these recipes are not only easy to cook but hardly take any time to cook. These nutritious and delicious recipes will further improve your overall health while following your chosen protocol of intermittent fasting. Making a dietary change is often easier than it sounds. You might be thinking it's all about changing your food habits. Well, intermittent fasting is so much more than that.

So, are you eager to learn more about intermittent fasting? If you want to feel more energetic and active than you ever did, intermittent fasting will leave you pleasantly surprised. Let us get started immediately!

Intermittent Fasting 101

These days, many new illnesses have cropped up and humans are exposed to them. to. Most health problems we are facing these days are primarily associated with the consumption of poor diets and leading a predominantly sedentary lifestyle. By using the simple concept of fasting, you can reverse most of the damaging effects associated with the above-mentioned factors. The concept of fasting is not new. It is a time-tested tradition and has been a part of human life since the dawn of civilization and even before. Fasting is commonly practiced for medical as well as spiritual reasons.

An unfortunate notion most have about fasting is it is synonymous with starvation. You cannot make fasting a part of your daily life unless you keep an open mind to it. It's essential to understand that fasting is not the same as starvation. Starvation is seldom voluntary. Fasting, on the other hand, is the voluntary abstinence from eating. When you fast, you are voluntarily preventing yourself from eating any solid foods or calories. Also, starvation is harmful, whereas fasting is a great way to improve your overall health. Fasting is a common practice in most cultures and religions across the world. Did you know that the father of modern science, Hippocrates, was a staunch supporter of regular fasts? A common treatment prescribed by him was fasting and drinking apple cider vinegar on an empty stomach to improve one's overall health. A popular saying by Hippocrates suggests that eating when sick is the surest way to fester the illness. If you take a moment and think about it, this makes sense. Most of us lose our appetite when unwell. This is our body's natural way of telling us we need to take a break and give our digestive system a much-needed breather. You might

have noticed that you lose the inclination to eat when you are down with the flu! Other famous Greek thinkers such as Aristotle, Plato, and Plutarch supported the notion of regular fast. They believed fasting was not just a preventive technique but a cure as well. The human body is extremely intuitive and powerful, but we don't give it the credit it deserves. It is capable of healing and repairing itself from the inside. Most of us forget that Fasting is embedded into our genetics.

What is Intermittent Fasting ?

To understand the concept of intermittent fasting, differentiating between fed and fasted states is important. Your body exists in either of these states at all times. It cannot exist in both these states simultaneously. Humans have come a long way. We now have additional comforts, technologies, and innovations at our disposal that would baffle our early ancestors. Our lives have become quite convenient and comfortable. Unfortunately, most of the health problems humanity is suffering from these days are associated with this convenience and comfort. Most of us are guilty of consuming unhealthy foods rich in calories and devoid of nutrients. We are also used to snacking constantly.

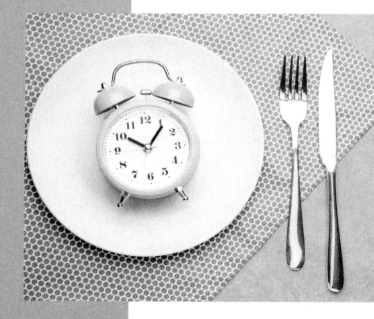

Whenever you eat, your body is in a fed state. During this, the internal mechanisms work to convert the food consumed into energy.

Most of the available energy is diverted to the digestive system to facilitate the digestion, absorption, and assimilation of the food consumed. However, your body does not immediately utilize all the energy it produces. Instead, only a portion of it is used while the rest is stored. Are you wondering how the extra energy is stored? They are stored in the form of fat deposits. Think of these reserves of fat as your body's individual savings account for a rainy day.

Now, let's move on to the next concept – fasted state. This is the opposite of the fed state. You are in a fasted state when you voluntarily or involuntarily abstain from eating. During a fasted state, your body is forced to start utilizing its existing and stored reserves of energy for sustenance. Your body doesn't have any other means of sustaining itself apart from utilizing the stored fats.

The only time most of us are in this state is when we are asleep. When you are asleep, your body is utilizing its existing reserves, and once they are exhausted, it starts using fats stored within.

Are you wondering what intermittent fasting means? The concept of I.F. is based on the idea of oscillating between fasting and fed states. To do this, you will need to fast for a specific period, eat, and then fast again, and so on. By doing this, your old cells have more time to be replaced with newborn, healthy ones.

Benefits of Intermittent Fasting

Intermittent fasting is one of the most fruitful and well-rounded diets available these days. Most benefits it offers are due to cellular changes that occur when your body shifts from a fed to a fasted state. During this, it finally gets a break from focusing most of its energy on digestive functions and instead concentrates on the other processes. One such process

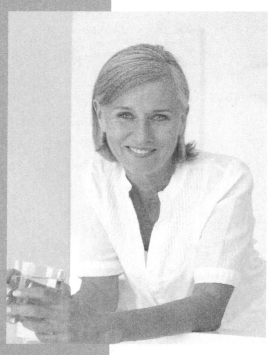

is autophagy. Autophagy refers to a self-cleaning mechanism where healthy ones cannibalize unhealthy, malfunctioning, and old cells to make more room. This helpful process is associated with a variety of benefits such as increased production of human growth hormone, better digestive health, improved skin health, cellular regeneration, and longevity are associated with autophagy. Autophagy is also responsible for detoxifying your body from the inside. So, any damage caused by excess toxic buildup is automatically reversed while following the intermittent fasting protocols.

Your blood sugar levels are also stabilized when you start following intermittent fasting. If you pause for a second to think about it, this makes perfect sense. Your body does not need any insulin unless you consume foods that have to be converted into glucose. Similarly, if your body cannot produce the required insulin, glucose levels start increasing. This also occurs when your body has developed insulin resistance. When you don't eat anything, and your body is in a fasted state, you won't need insulin. It means you don't have to worry about any spikes in blood sugar levels. In this way, fasting regularly can help improve your internal metabolism and reduce the risk of diabetes and help manage your blood sugar levels.

Acetoacetic acid
A product of Ketoacidosis

The production of human growth hormone or HGH usually declines with age. The production of this essential hormone reduces once you are above 50. This crucial hormone is responsible for regulating your metabolism, muscle and bone development and health, and your body composition. When you shift to intermittent fasting, the production of HGH automatically increases, resulting in an improvement in your overall health. In the next chapter, you will learn more about all the different benefits women over 50 can enjoy by shifting to intermittent fasting.

7 Myths About IF

1: SKIPPING BREAKFAST IS UNDESIRABLE

Breakfast is said to be the most important meal of the day. Well, it turns out this is nothing but a myth. Skipping breakfast is not harmful to your health. You can decide whether you want to eat or skip breakfast. When you are asleep, your body is in a fasted state and is utilizing its internal reserves of energy for sustenance. It will keep doing this until the feeding window. Your calorie consumption increases whenever you eat. If you skip a meal, calorie intake will reduce. This is needed for weight loss and maintenance. So, stop worrying that skipping breakfast will result in weight gain or it will harm your health.

2: WEIGHT LOSS – EATING SMALL MEALS

A common misconception is that eating small meals is needed for weight loss. Previously, you were introduced to the two natural states of the human body– fed and fasted. If you are constantly eating, you are in a fed state. The benefits of intermittent fasting cannot be reaped if you aren't in a fasted state. Also, the total number of calories you consume matters. Let us assume your daily calorie intake is 2000 calories. You can easily consume three large meals or five small meals within this limit. However, if you don't fast and keep eating, your body doesn't get a chance to reset its internal systems.

3: INTERMITTENT FASTING INCREASES RISK OF EATING DISORDERS

Intermittent fasting is one of the healthiest dietary protocols available these days. If you are not severely restricting your calorie consumption or starving, the risk of eating disorders is quite low. That said, if you have a history of eating disorders or are at the moment recovering from one, it's not the ideal time to follow any diet. Unless you are fully recovered, do not attempt any diet. Also, don't fail to consult your doctor or healthcare provider before opting for a dietary overhaul.

4: NUTRIENT DEFICIENCIES ARE ASSOCIATED WITH INTERMITTENT FASTING

You don't have to worry about nutrient deficiencies if you are carefully following the protocols of IF. Intermittent fasting doesn't mean you aren't allowed to eat or shouldn't eat if you don't pay attention to the foods consumed, the risk of nutritional deficiencies increases. Consuming nutrient-dense and wholesome ingredients during the eating window will reduce the risk of nutritional deficiencies. This is also a reason why making healthy food choices is crucial. In these subsequent chapters, you will be introduced to a variety of ingredients that should be added to your daily diet. If you are still worried about developing a nutrition deficiency, consult your healthcare provider and take a nutrient supplement as prescribed.

5: OVEREATING IS A SIDE EFFECT OF INTERMITTENT FASTING

Making healthy dietary choices and regulating your appetite are simple things that you have complete control over. By opting for fiber-rich and nutrient-dense foods, the chances of overheating are reduced. While your body is getting used to intermittent fasting protocols, chances are you might overeat a little. Once you are used to fasting, this does not happen. To further reduce the risk of overeating, ensure that you have healthy and nutritious meals to consume after the fasting period. This reduces the urge to binge on unhealthy foods.

6: MUSCLE LOSS IS A SIDE EFFECT OF I.F.

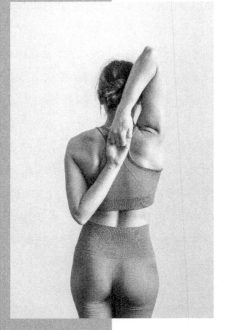

Periodic fasting does not result in muscle loss. As long as an internal resource of energy is present within your body, fasting is fine. This, coupled with the consumption of wholesome meals, means you don't have to worry about muscle loss at all. Self-cannibalization occurs only when your body has exhausted all the reserves of energy present. By adding a little exercise to your daily routine and paying attention to the meals consumed, you can maintain muscles while losing weight.

7: THE BRAIN CANNOT SUSTAIN WITHOUT CONSTANT SNACKING

A common myth is that the brain cannot sustain itself without a constant supply of carbs. This is one of the reasons why most believe constant snacking is the only way to maintain their cognitive well-being and functioning. Well, you don't have to worry about any reduction in your cognitive health while shifting to intermittent fasting. This is because the human body is adaptive and included. It is a self-sustaining machine that's capable of taking care of its needs and requirements. Certain parts of the brain require glucose for their functioning. That said, you don't have to constantly eat carbs to give your body the glucose it needs. A process known as gluconeogenesis helps produce glucose from proteins in the absence of carbs.

Intermittent fasting doesn't promote starvation. As long as you consume healthy and wholesome meals during the eating window, your body gets all the nutrients needed to complete normal functions. If you feel lightheaded or experience fatigue, it probably means you aren't eating enough during the eating window.

Not that you have gone through all the information discussed in this chapter, chances are you already feel quite good about trying intermittent fasting. Intermittent fasting is in no way harmful and, instead, is a great way to improve your overall health and well-being.

Intermittent Fasting After Turning 50

WE ALL GO THROUGH DIFFERENT STAGES IN LIFE. WE GO THROUGH CHILDHOOD, ADULTHOOD, AND OLD AGE.

A variety of physiological changes accompanies this transition from one stage to another. Menopause comes with a variety of physiological changes with far-reaching effects. Expect plenty of changes as you reach the big five-oh! The good news is that following intermittent fasting makes it easier to get accustomed to these changes.

Changes That Women Experience Once They Hit the Big Five-Oh!

A reduction in the production of certain hormones in a woman's body causes menopause. So, what are all the changes that occur within your body during menopause? Pretty much all the systems within your body are affected by menopause, including the reproductive system, endocrine system, skeletal system, cardiovascular system, nervous system, muscular system, and immune system.

Reproductive System

One of the major parts of your body affected by menopause is the reproductive organ. During the perimenopause period, the menstruation cycle becomes irregular, and your period might come and go without a fixed timetable. Until the period stops altogether, you don't hit menopause. At this stage, the production of eggs used for fertilization seizes. Menstruation occurs when the body sheds the unfertilized egg every month. Other parts of the reproductive system, such as the absence of clotting of cervical mucus mid-cycle, are usually associated with ovulation. A side effect of menopause is it harms your sex drive. The overall dryness of the vagina and lack of libido might be a setback because the naturally produced lubricants in the vagina also stop during menopause. However, this isn't necessarily a permanent change. Using an over-the-counter lubricant and consulting an OB-GYN for pharmaceutical assistance can reduce the severity of the symptoms experienced during menopause.

Nervous System

Whenever there are any hormonal changes in the body, it affects your overall mood. The same stands true during menopause as well. There will be days when you feel like you're at the top of the world and others when you are down in the dumps. You can also experience extreme mood swings causing irritability. Some women also experience anxiety and depression. According to the research undertaken by Freeman et al. (2006), menopause can be a trigger for anxiety and depression. Even if you have no previous history of any mental health conditions, menopause can change things up.

If the symptoms of depression or anxiety continue for a couple of weeks, you should seek professional help immediately.

You might also experience brain fog or poor memory during menopause. The reason for this is not yet known, but it seems to be a common symptom most women experience during menopause. As you age, memory loss is quite common. That said, it is not yet clear whether there is a correlation between menopause and memory.

Endocrine System

The endocrine system is responsible for regulating hormones associated with reproduction. Estrogen and progesterone are essential reproductive hormones, and a drastic reduction in their production causes some unpleasant physical symptoms such as hot flashes. This is one of the most common talked about side effects of menopause that occur due to the lack of estrogen. Women can experience hot flashes for up to a couple of years after menopause as well. A sudden feeling that your body is heating up and excessive sweating are all collectively known as hot flashes. They can occur at any time during the day and can last for a couple of seconds or even minutes at a time.

The simplest way to prevent and manage hot flashes is by making simple lifestyle changes such as avoiding hot beverages and caffeinated drinks. Apart from this, mindfulness techniques such as meditation also come in handy. During menopause, your body starts preserving more energy, which means calories and fat are not exhausted as they used to be. This can result in unnecessary weight gain. The chances of menopausal women gaining fat, especially in their abdominal region, increase. By tacking on a little exercise to your day-to-day routine, you can reduce the risk of this!

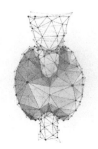

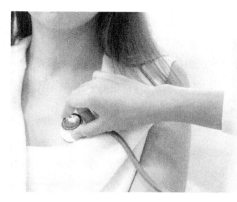

Cardiovascular System

Estrogen plays an essential role in the health of your cardiovascular system. It has a cardioprotective effect. Menopause is characterized by a reduction in the production of estrogen. The risk of cardiovascular disorders can increase during and after menopause, according to the findings of (Zhao et al. 2018). Estrogens also regulates your levels of cholesterol. Suppose the levels of estrogen reduce, the levels of cholesterol increase. This, in turn, increases the risk of heart attacks or strokes. Roelfsema (2018) also found that the hormones produced in the body during menopause can highly increase the risk of cardiovascular pathologies. This is one of the reasons why hormone replacement therapy is recommended for counteracting some of these damaging effects of menopause.

Benefits of IF for Women Over 50

Intermittent fasting is one of the elite diets these days. A great thing about IF is that it is ideal for all adults! All the benefits of this diet are backed by solid science and research. Also, this diet is proven to improve the health of women over 50!

Weight Loss and Maintenance

Intermittent fasting has become quite popular these days, especially with those who want to lose weight or maintain their weight loss. A calorie deficit is a precondition for weight loss. If your calorie intake is lower than calorie consumption, a calorie deficit is created. Short-term fasts such as the ones prescribed by intermittent fasting increase the production of a helpful neurotransmitter known as norepinephrine, according to the findings of (Zauner et al. 2000). This neurotransmitter activates your body's fat-burning mechanism. By following the protocols of intermittent fasting, you can attain your weight loss objectives according to a review presented by (Tinsley et al. 2015).

Increased Growth Hormone

Several hormones are responsible for your overall health and body's functioning. The human growth hormone (HGH) is one such hormone. With age, the production of this hormone declines naturally in the body. A reduction in this hormone can severely affect your overall health and well-being. The production of growth hormone increases when you follow the

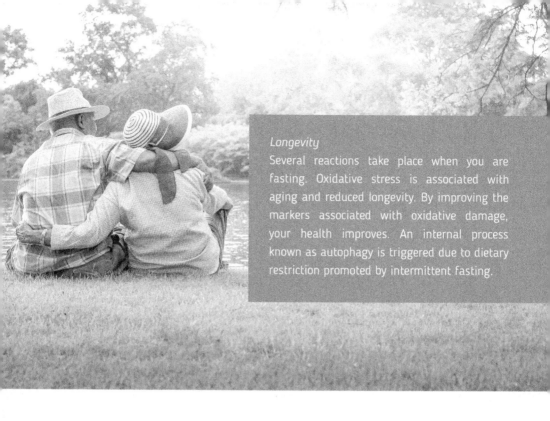

protocols of intermittent fasting, according to the research conducted by (Rasmussen et al. 1995). Similar results will also be obtained by another study undertaken by (Ho et al. 1988). This important hormone helps maintain your muscle strength, body temperature, kidney functioning, and stamina as well. It is also important for weight management. Glucose metabolism increases while following the protocols of intermittent fasting due to HGH production, according to (Moller et al. 1991). A decline in HGH production increases the risk of obesity, according to a study conducted by (Rasmussen 2010). Fasting for even 10 hours at a stretch causes a significant spike in the production of HGH, according to (Salgin et al. 2012).

These claims are also backed by another study (Hartman et al. 1992). When the insulin and blood sugar levels are stabilized in the body, it automatically increases the production of HGH.

Better Cardiovascular Health

There is a direct correlation between heart health and fasting. This could be due to how the cholesterol and blood sugar levels are balanced during fasting. The presence of low-density lipoprotein, commonly dubbed as bad cholesterol or LDL, reduces when you follow any of the protocols of intermittent fasting discussed in the previous chapter. Apart from this, intermittent fasting also improves your body's ability to regulate blood sugar levels on its own and diminish the risk of diabetes. This, coupled with its weight loss benefits, reduces the risk factors associated with cardiovascular disorders.. Dong et al. (2020) noted that intermittent fasting helps improve heart health.

Balanced Blood Sugar Levels

A hormone known as insulin is produced by the pancreas whenever any food is consumed. This hormone breaks down the food and transforms it into an easily absorbable
source of energy known as glucose. Different cells in the body utilize this glucose thus produced. The level of blood sugar is directly associated with insulin production and its effectiveness. Type-2 diabetes occurs when your body is incapable of producing insulin needed for regulating your blood sugar levels.

If your body starts developing resistance toward insulin, more insulin is needed to perform its usual function. These two conditions cause diabetes. The research undertaken by Heilbronn et al. (2005) shows that intermittent fasting helps restabilize blood sugar levels. Similar findings were also obtained from a pilot study conducted by (Arnason et al. 2017). Insulin resistance reduces when you follow calorie restrictions. A wonderful thing about intermittent fasting is your calorie intake reduces even if you are not consciously counting every calorie consumed. By reducing insulin resistance, your body's ability to manage its blood sugar levels improves. This ensures the glucose present within is circulating and entering cells from the bloodstream efficiently. A combination of both these factors helps table your blood sugar levels. This, in turn, reduces the risk of type II diabetes.

Reduced Risk of Alzheimer's and Better Cognitive Health

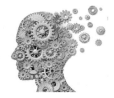

A common medical remedy prescribed by ancient Greeks was fasting. They believed fasting promotes cognitive functioning. It turns out they were onto something quite valuable. When it comes to improving your cognitive health, fasting helps. The findings of Li et al. (2013) suggest that short-term fasting enhances functioning and the structure of the brain. Most results are from animal models, but the positive benefits and promising potential of intermittent fasting for improving brain health cannot be ignored. Intermittent fasting promotes the creation of new neural cells and networks in mice, according to (Lee et al. 2000). Intermittent fasting improves cognitive functioning, according to the findings of (Tajes et al.(2010). Alzheimer's is associated with cognitive decline and aging. Intermittent fasting coupled with mindful calorie restriction can reduce the risk of cognitive decline and improve the brain's health, according to (Martin et al. 2009).

Regulating Inflammation

Your body has an internal defense system known as the immune system. The primary role of the immune system is to maintain your overall health and fight any infections or disease-causing pathogens present within. It does this by triggering the first line of defense known as inflammation. Inflammation is important for maintaining your overall health and well-being. That said, when left unregulated, it becomes detrimental to health. This natural immune response should stop once the threat is eliminated, and the inflammation must subside. If it persists, it results in a condition known as chronic inflammation. In this, the immune system mistakenly attacks healthy cells and even itself resulting in significant internal damage. Chronic inflammation is associated with severe health problems and even painful conditions such as rheumatoid arthritis, multiple sclerosis and increases the risk of cardiovascular disorders.

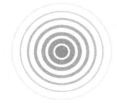

inflammatory markers in the body then use both intermittent fasting methods, according to the results obtained by (Faris et al. 2012). Similar results were also noticed by (Aksungar et al. 2007). Any diet that creates similar results like the ones prescribed by intermittent fasting reduces inflammation, according to the results of an animal study undertaken by (Choi et al. 2016). This comes in handy to treat multiple sclerosis and other inflammatory conditions, according to these researchers.

Reduces the Risk of Cancer

There's some ongoing research that suggests the potential of intermittent fasting to help minimize the risk of certain types of cancer. It's important to know most of these results are from animal and test-tube studies. For instance, according to one study by Rocha et al. (2002), it was noted that intermittent fasting restricts the growth and formation of tumors and growth of tumors in rats. Lee et al. (2013) conducted a test-tube study to understand the role of intermittent fasting and tumors. It was noted that intermittent fasting delayed the onset of tumors. Researchers of the study also noticed this effect: it's quite similar to the ones obtained by chemotherapy on cancerous cells. These results are quite promising. That said, extensive research is further needed to fully understand how intermittent fasting can help reduce the risk of certain types of cancer and too much.

The findings of Chiofalo et al. (2017) suggest that intermittent fasting can be used as a complementary therapy for treating PCOS. PCOS is associated with weight gain and insulin resistance. Both these symptoms can be managed by following intermittent fasting. Insulin resistance also reduces the presence of male sexual hormones in women, .

Skin Health

What you eat reflects on your skin. If you want healthy skin, you need to start paying attention to your diet. Inflammation harms your skin health. For instance, dermatitis, acne, and other skin problems are inflammatory conditions. As mentioned, intermittent fasting helps reduce inflammation. This, in turn, improves your skin health. Oxidative damage speeds up aging. By reversing oxidative damage and inflammation, intermittent fasting helps improve your skin health. If you want glowing and supple skin, start following any of the protocols of intermittent fasting discussed in the previous section.

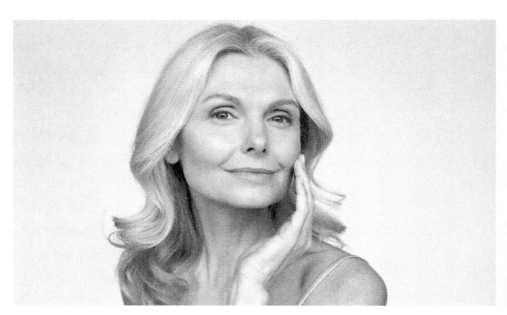

This, coupled with a healthy diet devoid of unhealthy carbs and processed foods, further benefits your skin. Instead of splurging on expensive skincare, start concentrating on your diet!

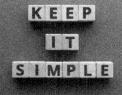

Effect on Circadian Rhythm

This circadian rhythm is responsible for regulating your body's internal sleep-wake cycles. Think of it like an internal alarm clock responsible for keeping you awake during the day and asleep at night. Unfortunately, this rhythm can be harmed by a variety of lifestyle factors ranging from extreme stress to hectic schedules, poor sleep patterns, and unhealthy eating habits. If you eat late at night, your ability to sleep is also hampered. This not only increases the risk of diabetes and obesity but harms the circadian rhythm as well.

A wonderful thing about the intermittent fasting protocols is they restrict the eating window. Suppose you eat early in the night, your ability to fall asleep at an appropriate time increases. When you sleep on time, it becomes easier to wake up early. If you keep following this schedule, your internal body clock is once again realigned. According to the findings of Almeneessier et al. (2018), intermittent fasting can help regulate your body's sleep-wake cycle. So, if you are struggling to sleep at night or wake up early, it's time to change your diet. Add a little exercise to your daily routine, and it will further improve your ability to sleep at night.

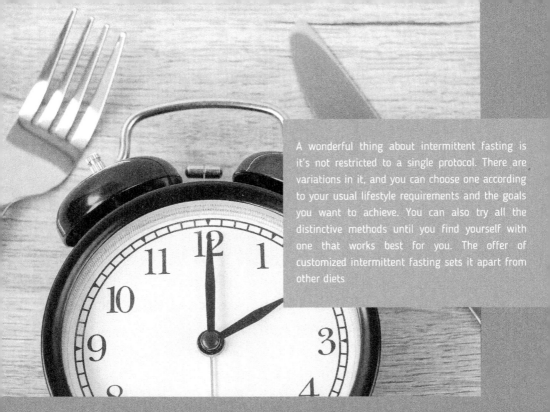

A wonderful thing about intermittent fasting is it's not restricted to a single protocol. There are variations in it, and you can choose one according to your usual lifestyle requirements and the goals you want to achieve. You can also try all the distinctive methods until you find yourself with one that works best for you. The offer of customized intermittent fasting sets it apart from other diets

Different Methods of Intermittent Fasting

5:2 Method

The 5:2 method is an incredibly simple variation of intermittent fasting. If you have never tried fasting before, start with this before making your way to the other options discussed in this section. According to this method, you need to fast for only two days and eat like you ordinarily do for the rest of the days of the week. Even on the days you are fasting, you are allowed to consume between 500–600 calories.

For instance, eat like you normally do on all days of the week except Tuesdays and Fridays. On these two days, you will need to restrict your calorie intake to 500-600 calories. Within this calorie limit, you can consume two small meals or one large meal according to your choice. You can fast on any day that you want. The only condition is you should never fast on two consecutive days. Pick the two busiest days of your week and turn them into your fasting days. If your mind is distracted, fasting becomes quite easy.

Eat – Stop – Eat Protocol

Once you get into the groove of fasting and are comfortable with the above-mentioned method, try this protocol. The only rule for following the eat–stop–eat protocol is you should not fast on two consecutive days. Apart from the fasting days, you can pretty much follow your regular diet on all the other days. The idea of this protocol is to fast for 24-hours at a stretch and not any longer. This is the reason why you should never fast on two consecutive days. For instance, if the fast starts on Monday night at 9, you will need to fast until 9:00 PM on Tuesday. Yes, this is as simple as that is. If you are fasting on Monday and Tuesday, your next fast shouldn't be until Thursday. If you fast for longer than 24-hours, it will shift your body into starvation mode and will prevent the benefits associated with intermittent fasting.

You can consume no-calorie beverages such as unsweetened tea or coffee.

16:8 Fasting

This is one of the most commonly followed methods of intermittent fasting. In this method, you need to fast for 16-hours daily while the eating window is restricted to 8-hours. So, all the calories you eat and drink need to be restricted to this 8-hour window. The cycle can be customized according to your liking. You don't have to fast daily. If you want, you can fast for a couple of days every week until you feel more comfortable. This method has become one of the favorite intermittent fasting techniques, especially am

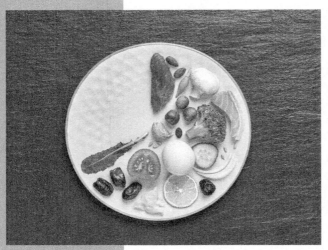

ong those who want to achieve weight loss and fitness goals. During the fasting window,you're not supposed to consume any calories, and this is the one rule you shouldn't forget. Also, the fasting window should be completed at a stretch. For instance, if you stop eating on Monday at 9 PM, you will need to fast until 1 PM on Tuesday. By doing this, you have fasted for 16-hours, and you can eat between 1-9 PM on Tuesday. Most of the fasting window goes away during the nighttime, making it easier to fast on the following day. Think of this protocol as a mere extension of your sleeping period. Once again, you are free to customize the eating and fasting windows according to your convenience. During the fasting window, you're not supposed to consume any calories, and that his is the one rule you shouldn't forget. Also, the fasting window should be completed at a stretch. For instance, if you stop eating on Monday at 9 PM, you will need to fast until 1 PM on Tuesday. By doing this, you have fasted for 16-hours, and you can eat between 1-9 PM on Tuesday. Most of the fasting window goes away during the nighttime, making it easier to fast on the following day. If you sleep for 7-hours, the fasting window is only 9-hours! Think of this protocol as a mere extension of your sleeping period. Once again, you are free to customize the eating and fasting windows according to your convenience.

14:10 Fasting

In this method of intermittent fasting, you will be fasting for 14-hours daily while the eating window is restricted to 10-hours. If you want, you can fast daily or even on alternate days. As mentioned, all the methods of IF can be customized according to your needs and requirements. Rest easy because intermittent fasting doesn't have to clash with your usual lifestyle. You can eat regularly between the hours of 10:00 AM until 8:00 PM. After 8:00 PM, the fasting window starts and extends until 10:00 AM on the following day. When you do this, you are effectively fasting for 14-hours. It is as simple as that.

20:4 Fasting

This protocol of intermittent fasting is also known as the warrior diet. In this method, the eating window is restricted to only 4-hours. You will have to fast for 20-hours and eat within the 4-hour window. You can consume one healthy and hearty meal within this timeframe that has the required energy to keep going through the fasting period. There is also a variation of the warrior diet. If you want, you can consume healthy foods such as vegetables, nuts, dairy items, and even hard-boiled eggs during the day. However,

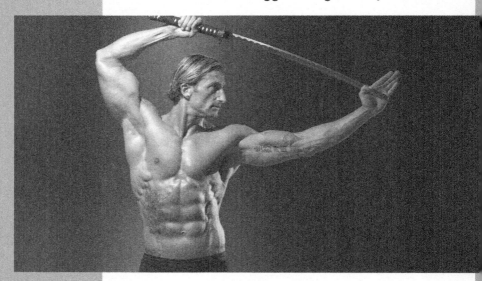

ensure you don't consume too many calories during the day and then binge at night. Following this diet becomes quite easy as long as you consume these organic foods in limited quantities and non-calorie beverages. If you are following a strict 20:4 approach, then you cannot consume any calories during the 20-hour fasting window.

Hitching a Ride on the I.F. Bandwagon

INTERMITTENT FASTING PLACES SUCH A GREAT EMPHASIS ON WHEN YOU EAT INSTEAD OF WHAT YOU EAT. THAT SAID, CERTAIN FOODS WILL HELP IMPROVE YOUR HEALTH WHILE OTHERS MIGHT WORK AGAINST IT.

For instance, if you fast all day long and end the fast by snacking on unhealthy junk and processed foods, all your efforts go to waste. After all, what is the point of eating ice cream and chips for dinner after fasting for 16-hours? Even though there are no dietary rules in intermittent fasting, it's important to consume a well-balanced diet.

After going through all the different benefits of intermittent fasting, chances are you are extremely excited to get started with this diet. Here are some suggestions and helpful advice that will come in handy while shifting to intermittent fasting.

During the Fast

The only rule of fasting is to ensure that you don't consume many calories. The moment you consume calories, your body shifts from a fasted to a fed state. To avoid this, become mindful of what you consume during the fasting window.

Apple Cider Vinegar

Having apple cider vinegar during the fasting window will work wonders for your overall health. It is a zero-calorie beverage that helps rebalance the internal pH levels while reducing hunger pangs. It also stabilizes the electrolyte levels. Apple cider vinegar is believed to improve the health and functioning of the immune and digestive systems. It also offers a quick boost to your body's fat-burning abilities. It is also a rich source of different minerals such as magnesium, iron, and potassium. You can have up to two tablespoons of apple cider vinegar daily. It is said that this wonderful ingredient improves skin health as well. Pour slowly some apple cider vinegar into a glass of warm water and sip this concoction to keep hunger away. Alternatively, consume it without any water too!

Herbal Teas

Drinking herbal teas during the fasting window not only elevates hunger pangs but can quickly reenergize you as well. The only rule is to remember that it must be unsweetened. You cannot add any natural sweeteners, including stevia or honey. Also, you cannot add any form of diary to your cup of tea. A freshly brewed cup of chamomile tea can instantly calm your mind, or peppermint tea can reenergize you. Experiment with different blends and combinations of herbal teas according to your needs. When in doubt, having a cup of freshly brewed green tea will do the trick. Green tea is a powerhouse of antioxidants that reduce inflammation and improve your body's ability to metabolize fats.

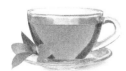

Baking Soda

Baking soda is commonly used in cooking and baking. This ingredient can also be consumed during the fasting window. Baking soda helps regulate your pH

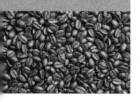

levels that change during the fasting window. Take a glass of water and add one teaspoon of baking soda to it. Mix it thoroughly and drink. . Drink this to instantly elevate your energy levels and tackle any hunger pangs. Baking soda or sodium bicarbonate helps replenish any of the sodium your body loses during the fasting phase. This ensures your electrolyte levels are well-balanced because ketosis has a diuretic effect. By neutralizing all this, it becomes easier to get through the fasting window.

Glauber's Salts

A simple way to improve your body's metabolism while getting through the fasting window is by drinking a glass of water mixed with Glauber's salt. Glauber's salt is known as sodium sulfate decahydrate. It is fit for daily consumption and is believed to restabilize the electrolyte levels. When your electrolyte levels are well-balanced, the chances of dehydration reduce drastically. Since dehydration is one of the leading causes of hunger and headaches associated with fasting, you can do away with it by adding some Glauber's salts. Remember, you should not consume more than 20 grams of it on any given day because consuming too much of it can cause diarrhea. It is a mild laxative and improves digestion while relieving constipation when consumed in moderation. Add a teaspoon of these salts to a glass of water for consumption. Have this whenever you feel hungry.

Ending the Fast

While following most protocols of intermittent fasting, you need to strictly adhere to the eating and fasting windows prescribed by them. How you break, the fast is as important as what you do during the fasting window. Even if it sounds simple, there will be days when your motivation levels falter. There will be times when regardless of how hard you try, following the fast becomes quite difficult. This is why you should always have a plan in mind about how you want to go about ending the fast. If you don't plan, the risk of giving up on the diet increases.

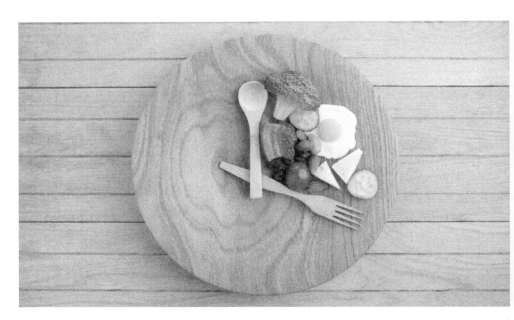

Different desirable changes take place within your body during fasting time. An important change is your body shifts into a state of ketosis, especially if you are fasting for anywhere between 10 and 16-

You can drink bone or vegetable broth to end the fast. Bone broth is a superfood rich in essential nutrients and electrolytes. Once again, these ingredients stimulate the production of essential digestive enzymes. It also prepares your gut to absorb nutrients from the food you will consume during the eating window. Your body is in a self-cleaning mode while fasting. Essentially, it is in a state of rest. Drinking bone or vegetable broth, water mixed with honey and lime juice, or some apple cider vinegar acts as a much-needed warm-up before exercise. If your fast extends over 10-hours, following the above-mentioned tips will help.

hours. During ketosis, the ketones produced by the liver give your body the energy it needs for sustenance. This increases the stress on the digestive system. How you break the fast plays a significant role in the stress on your digestive system. If you are not careful, the excess stress caused by bingeing on foods as soon as a diet ends can trigger inflammation, which is associated with weight gain and a reduction in the efficiency of the immune system. To avoid all this, you need to have a plan in place to break the fast.

One of the safest and an effective means to an end fast is by drinking a little apple cider vinegar. As mentioned, this wonderful ingredient helps restore pH levels in the gut while neutralizing harmful bacteria present within the digestive tract. Because it is a calorie-free ingredient, make it a point to consume it during the fast and as soon as it ends. Adding a little cinnamon and lemon juice helps mask the flavor of raw apple cider vinegar. Adding a pinch of salt to it also helps restabilize the electrolyte levels in your body. Drink this mixture and give your body about 30 minutes to get acclimatized to producing digestive juices. When you do this, your gut starts preparing itself for the food you are about to consume. Alternatively, you can also drink a glass of warm water mixed with lemon juice and honey. The citric acid present in these ingredients stimulates the digestive enzymes and acts as a warm-up exercise for the gut.

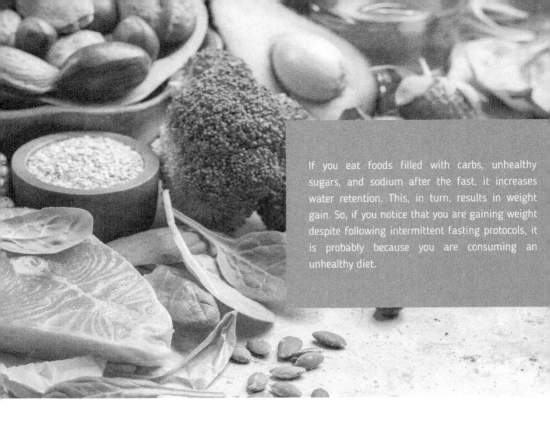

If you eat foods filled with carbs, unhealthy sugars, and sodium after the fast, it increases water retention. This, in turn, results in weight gain. So, if you notice that you are gaining weight despite following intermittent fasting protocols, it is probably because you are consuming an unhealthy diet.

What to Eat During the Eating Window?

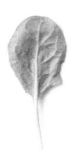

Unless you are following the 5:2 method or the eat-stop-eat protocol of intermittent fasting, getting accustomed to the idea of fasting daily takes time. You not only have to prepare your body for ending the fast, but you must concentrate on the diet you consume after the fast ends too. If you want to take advantage of intermittent fasting, consuming a well-balanced nutritious diet cannot be overlooked.

Insulin is needed to promote the transportation of essential nutrients from one cell to another within the body. Any dramatic spike or fluctuation in insulin levels is caused by the consumption of carbs and sugars. This can make you feel quite drowsy and lethargic. So, the first meal you consume, after the fast ends, shouldn't have a high glycemic index. A low glycemic meal enables your body to stay in the semi-fasted state for longer and reduces any dramatic fluctuations in blood sugar levels.

All the health benefits offered by fasting become redundant if you eat foods with a high glycemic index during the eating window. Any food that increases the glycogen reserves results in fat accumulation. If you want to eat fresh fruits, opt for ones that are low in sugars and rich in dietary fibers, such as different types of berries, melons, and apples. If you start becoming mindful of what you eat after the fast ends, the chances of maximizing the benefits offered by intermittent fasting automatically increase.

There aren't any calorie restrictions or strict dietary restrictions per se in intermittent fasting. That said, when following the 5:2 diet, you cannot exceed 600 calories on the fasting days. Except for this fasting protocol, you don't have to trouble yourself about calorie counting on the other methods. Once again, it's important to be prudent about the food choices you make while following this diet. After all, the aim of shifting to intermittent fasting is to enhance your overall health. If you keep overeating on unhealthy foods or foods rich in calories and devoid of nutrients, it does your body no favors whatsoever. Ensure that you plan the meals such that your body gets its daily dose of nutrients. Follow the different intermittent fasting friendly recipes given in this book, and it will ensure your body gets all the nutrients that are required.

Certain foods are better suited for intermittent fasting than others. As mentioned, consumption of nutrient-devoid carbs and sugars is harmful to your overall health and well-being. Most problems humanity faces these days are due to a combination of unhealthy diet and sedentary lifestyle. Here are some foods that will make a wonderful addition to your daily diet and will improve your nutritional intake without compromising on weight loss goals.

Fish

Adding naturally fatty fish and seafood to your daily diet is a wonderful idea. Fish is not only a rich source of heart-healthy omega-3 fatty acids but is a source of lean protein too. A combination of these two factors makes them an ideal fit for any weight loss and wholesome diet. Naturally fatty fish such as sardines, trout, salmon, mahi-mahi, cod, or mackerel will be good additions to your diet. You can consume up to 7-ounces of fatty fish daily. The Omega-3 fatty acids present in them promote cognitive functioning, counteract inflammation, and improve your heart's health. Lean protein reduces the stress on the digestive system. Whenever you decide to add any fish to your diet, opt for fish caught in the wild as much as possible instead of factory-farmed variants.

Leafy Vegetables

Swiss chard, kale, spinach, amaranth, rosella, and so on are all examples of leafy vegetables. Adding leafy vegetables to your diet gives your body its daily dose of minerals and vitamins along with dietary fiber and helpful antioxidants. Also, they are low-calorie food options. The low glycemic index of leafy greens makes them a wonderful addition to any meal you consume while following intermittent fasting.

Probiotics

The digestive system is home to millions of bacteria known as the gut microbiome. Don't worry because not all types of bacteria are disease-causing pathogens. Specific types of microbes found in the gut are responsible for promoting and maintaining digestive health and absorption of nutrients. Your digestive health automatically improves when the gut microbiome functions properly. This also reduces the chances of inflammation, digestive troubles, and other health conditions associated with poor gut health. This is where probiotics step into the picture. Probiotics refer to live microorganisms responsible for improving the health of the gut microbiome. Probiotics are fermented foods such as kimchi, yogurt, buttermilk, kombucha, and sauerkraut. Whenever possible, try to make these fermented foods at home instead of relying on store-bought variants. Most store-bought variants contain harmful sugars that you can easily avoid while making them at home.

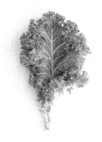

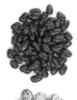

Avocados

Avocados seem to be the rage these days. Eating avocados is so much more than a fad or a trend. They are filled with heart-healthy fatty acids and are low in calories. They truly are a superfood. Also, the digestive fibers present in them promote gut health. It's also an incredible source of protein. Another wonderful thing about avocados is they can be easily incorporated into any meal of your choice. Whether it's a smoothie or a salad, adding avocados to your daily diet is quite simple. Their buttery and smooth flavor and texture can instantly elevate the flavor profile of any dish.

Legumes

Legumes contain vitamins, nutrients, and plenty of dietary fiber. The dietary fiber present in them not only promotes digestion but also enables better absorption of nutrients in the gut. Different types of legumes can be easily added to your diet. Also, they are a healthy source of complex carbs. Because they are rich in dietary fiber, the total carbs present in legumes are quite low when compared to carb-loaded food such as bread or pasta. Another advantage of adding legumes to your diet is they are quite filling. When you are full, it becomes quite difficult to overeat during the eating window. Since legumes are satiating, getting through the fasting window also becomes easier.

Whole Foods

While following any dietary regime, you must increase your consumption of whole foods. Simultaneously, avoid or significantly reduce the consumption of processed and prepackaged foods as much as you possibly can. Most prepackaged and processed foods available on the market these days are rich in undesirable calories without any helpful nutrients. If you load up on nutrient-devoid and calorie-rich foods, your hunger might be satiated for the time being, but it will be back with a vengeance. Consumption of such foods increases your calorie intake without the required nutrients. If weight or fat loss and maintenance is one of your objectives, increase your consumption of whole foods.

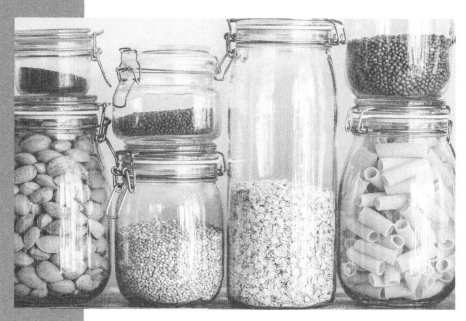

Berries

Berries are a wonderful addition to any diet. They are rich in a variety of antioxidants, dietary fiber, vitamin A, and vitamin C. Apart from it, they are low in calories too. From raspberries and blueberries to blackberries, strawberries, and even cherries, there are multiple options. Whether you want to enjoy a guilt-free dessert or have an antioxidants-rich smoothie, they can be easily incorporated into different meals. Batteries are known to promote the functioning of the immune system, regulate inflammation, and reverse the damage caused by oxidative stress. Berries can be consumed in that fresh or frozen form, depending on their availability.

Eggs

No diet is complete without eggs. Eggs are a rich source of dietary fats and healthy protein and have a low glycemic index. Add two eggs to your daily diet to increase the consumption of omega-3 fatty acids and protein. Another benefit of adding eggs to your diet is they are incredibly easy to cook with and versatile. Choose free-range or organic eggs whenever possible instead of the commercially farmed ones. The former is believed to be more nutritious than the latter.

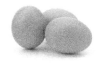

Apart from all the different food items mentioned until now, another important part of maintaining a healthy diet is keeping your body hydrated. To do this, you will need to drink at least eight glasses of water daily. You might need more depending on your rigorous level of activity and the usual environment.

6 STEPS TO START FOLLOWING I.F.

Now, let's get to the most important and interesting part of intermittent fasting – getting started with the diet! Here are some simple steps on suggestions you can use to get accustomed to the intermittent fasting way of life.

1 - Do Your Homework

Before you can get started, it's time to consider the intermittent fasting protocol that is right for you. You were introduced to different variations of intermittent fasting in the previous chapter. Carefully go through them, consider your usual lifestyle, and see which one

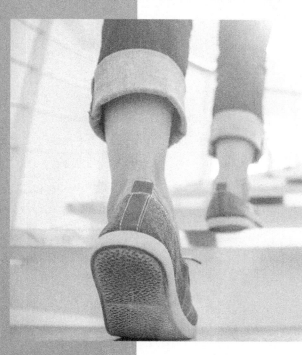

If you want, you can always follow the method of trial-and-error. Why don't you try different intermittent fasting protocols and see which one works well for you? If you don't mind a little extra effort right now, go ahead and do this.

Do you remember a childhood story in regards to the hare and tortoise? Just like the tortoise, remember that slow and steady wins the race. This should be your mantra when you are shifting to any diet, including intermittent fasting. Do not start this diet at once. Remember, think of a dietary change as a lifelong commitment. To make the diet sustainable, you need to start slow. If you are rushing into the diet, especially when you have no experience with fasting, it increases the chances of abandoning the diet altogether. Pace yourself and slowly transition to intermittent fasting. The idea of taking things slow is to gradually condition your mind to the concept of intermittent fasting. It's not just your body that needs to get used to the diet. Your attitude matters as well. Keep an open mind, try fasting for a brief period, and see what works for you.

would be an ideal fit for you. If the method of fasting clashes with your usual lifestyle or becomes too much for you to follow, the diet will not be sustainable. This is one of the reasons why selecting the ideal pattern of intermittent fasting is important. For instance, if you are not used to eating breakfast or prefer exercising early in the morning, the 16/8 method will work well. If you don't like the notion of fasting or are scared of it, you can start with the 5:2 method instead of the eat-stop-eat protocol. It is important to select a method that is comfortable for your body and mind. When you are on board with the fasting technique making this tired sustainable in the long run becomes easier.

2 – Gather the Tools

You will need some tools in place while making any dietary shift. Tools here don't mean a calorie counter. It could be something as simple as a meal plan, a recipe book, and a food journal. It becomes easier to follow the diet when you are aware of the food you will be eating. When you start following the etiquettes of intermittent fasting, you will become more conscious of your hunger cues. It will also help improve the relationship with food. For some good news, all the recipes you need to follow intermittent fasting protocols are discussed in this book. Carefully go through the recipes, the sample mean plan, and create a meal plan that works well for you.

Start maintaining a food diary or a journal. In this, make a note of everything you eat during the day. When you do this, you automatically become more aware of the food choices you are making. By eating healthier and nutrient-dense foods, your overall health will improve without piling on the additional calories. While doing this, you might also realize certain foods work well with your metabolism while others work against it.

3 - Start Slow

Let's assume that you are used to snacking constantly. In such instances, you will need to overcome this habit while following the protocols of intermittent fasting. Most protocols recommend a fasting period of anywhere between 10-24 hours. To get through such lengthy fasts, you need to overcome the habit of constant snacking. A simple way to do this is by slowly increasing the duration between the meals you consume. When you do this slowly, within a few weeks, you will get accustomed to not snacking altogether. Similarly, if your usual diet is rich in carbs, sugars, or even processed foods, shifting to intermittent fasting will take some time. Slowly increase your intake of healthy and wholesome ingredients, replace processed foods with whole foods, reduce your consumption of unhealthy carbs, and increase your intake of dietary fats and protein. When you do this, you are slowly conditioning your body toward a healthier diet. All the above-mentioned ingredients will naturally curb your appetite.

4 – Support System

We all need a little support at one point or another. When it comes to making dietary changes, this stands true. Your support system can include your friends, family members, loved ones, spouse, or anyone else of your choice. The idea of creating a support system is to share your goals and ideas of shifting to intermittent fasting. By doing this, you are automatically creating accountability and holding yourself accountable to others. There will be days when giving up on the diet seems easier than sticking to it, especially when you have no motivation to keep going. In such instances, your support system will come in handy. They will give you the needed motivation to keep going. Also, it helps when others check in to see how you are doing and enquire about the progress you make. This external sense of accountability will increase your motivation to stick by the promises you make.

If you want, you can also start this diet with someone else; think of it as a dieting buddy. When you know you aren't alone, getting through the fasting period, even when you don't feel like it, becomes easier. There is strength in numbers. Don't hesitate to reach out to others, especially on online platforms, who are following intermittent fasting protocols. Use online forums and social media platforms to connect with other similar-minded people. Sharing tips, advice, and experiences can be a motivating experience.

5- Protein is Important

While following any protocol of intermittent fasting, prioritize protein and complex carbs. These categories of foods increase satiety and give your body desired nutrients. Apart from this, they are relatively low in calories as well. Fasting will not always be easy. You need to mentally prepare yourself for it. There will be days when you don't feel like fasting, eating something unhealthy, or ending the fast quicker than

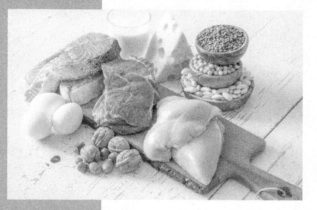 you should. On all such days, prioritize the consumption of proteins and complex carbs before eating anything else. For instance, if you want to have some ice cream, remind

yourself to fill up on your daily quota of protein and healthy carbs before moving on to ice cream. Chances are, by the time you are done eating the other foods, you will not have any space left for ice cream. This reduces the risk of overheating while ensuring that your body gets all the nutrients it needs before filling up on junk food. Concentrating on when you eat is important. At the same time, you should also pay a little attention to what you are eating. Do not compromise on portions while following any protocol of intermittent fasting. Remember, the food you consume during the eating window keeps your body

Previously, you were introduced to a list of ingredients you can consume during the fasting window, such as unsweetened black coffee and herbal tea, apple cider vinegar, Glauber's salts, and baking soda. By drinking these beverages, it becomes easier to regulate your hunger pangs. Apart from this, ensure to keep your mind thoroughly distracted or occupied during the fasting period. When you are preoccupied, it becomes easier to get through the fast without giving in to temptations.

fueled through the fasting period. If you don't eat anything when you are supposed to, then fasting will become difficult. Remember, earlier, you were introduced to the difference between fasting and starvation. Once your body shifts to starvation mode, all the benefits associated with intermittent fasting are nullified.. Instead, your body starts holding onto calories and fat to conserve energy. You want to avoid this and, therefore, do not scrimp on portions. That said, eat until you are full and no more. The only rule is to eat healthy and wholesome foods instead of processed ones.

6 – Dealing With Hunger

Perhaps the most common reason why dieting gets a bad rap is because of hunger. Dealing with hunger pangs is an important aspect of making any dietary change. The temptation to eat is quite powerful when you get hungry. Not just eat, your body usually craves carbs and sugar, two things you are not supposed to eat when hungry. To keep hunger pangs at bay, you should load up on complex carbs and protein, low-carb vegetables, and keep your body thoroughly hydrated. Apart from this, make it a point to eat until you are full. Understand that this is not the same as overeating. Learn to become mindful of your body's cues when it is getting hungry and eat accordingly.

Healthy Recipes for Intermittent Fasting

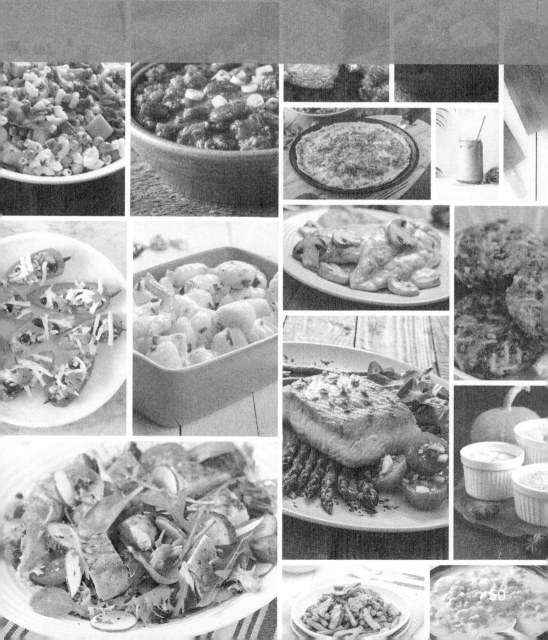

Turkey Sausage Frittata

 30 Minutes   20 minutes   4 servings   240 Kcal

INGREDIENTS

- 6 oz. ground breakfast turkey sausage
- 4 eggs
- ½ tsp. Himalayan pink salt
- 1 tsp. butter
- 1 bell pepper, thinly sliced
- ½ cup sour cream
- ½ tsp. black pepper
- 1 ounce Tillamook cheddar cheese, shredded

PER SERVING

Proteins: 16.7 g
Carbohidrates: 5.5 g
Fat: 16.7 g

DIRECTIONS

1. Whisk together sour cream, salt, eggs, and pepper in a blender until well combined.
2. Turn up the temperature of your oven to 350°F and turn on the oven.
3. Place a small ovenproof skillet over medium heat. Add butter and wait for a few seconds for the butter to melt.
4. Add bell pepper into the skillet and cook until tender. Transfer the bell pepper onto a plate.
5. Add sausage into the skillet and cook it until it turns brown. Break the meat into smaller pieces while stirring
6. Spread the meat on the bottom of the skillet. Scatter bell pepper over the meat.
7. Ladle the blended mixture over the meat and bell pepper in the skillet. Do not stir. Make sure the entire thing is covered with the blended mixture.
8. Turn off the heat and place the skillet into the oven. Start the timer for about 20 minutes.
9. Bake until the egg mixture is set. If you are using cheese, sprinkle cheese over the frittata during the last 3 – 4 minutes of baking.
10. Cut into 4 equal wedges and serve.

Matcha Smoothie

 5 Minutes   3 minutes   2 servings   75 Kcal

INGREDIENTS

- 6 ounces ground breakfast turkey sausage
- 4 eggs
- ½ tsp. Himalayan pink salt
- 1 teaspoon butter
- 1 bell pepper, thinly sliced
- ½ cup sour cream
- ½ tsp. black pepper
- 1 ounce Tillamook cheddar cheese, shredded

PER SERVING

Proteins: 4.2 g
Carbohidrates: 8.5 g
Fat: 1.2 g

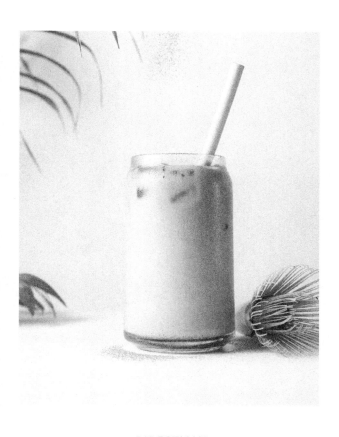

DIRECTIONS

1. In a fruit blender, combine together coconut milk, spinach, monk fruit sweetener, almonds, matcha powder, ice cubes, and blueberries until you get a smooth mixture.
2. Trickle or spoon it into glasses and serve.

Goat Cheese & Ham Omelet

 20 Minutes   5 minutes   2 servings 143 Kcal

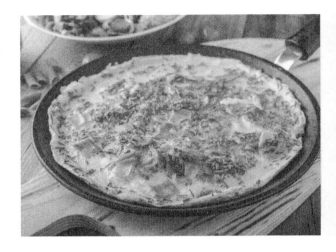

INGREDIENTS

- 8 large egg whites
- ¼ tsp. ground black pepper
- ¼ cup finely chopped green bell pepper
- ¼ cup crumbled goat cheese
- 4 tsp. water
- 2 slices deli ham, finely chopped
- ¼ cup finely chopped onion
- 1 tbsp. minced fresh parsley (optional)

PER SERVING

Proteins: 21.6 g
Carbohidrates: 5.0 g
Fat: 4.4g

DIRECTIONS

1. Place whites and water in a bowl and whisk until well incorporated.
2. Add ham, onion, bell pepper, and pepper and jumble until thoroughly blended.
3. Place a nonstick pan over medium-high heat. Spray the pan with cooking spray.
4. Pour half the omelet mixture into the pan. When the omelet is cooked, scatter half the cheese on one half of the omelet.
5. Fold the other half of the omelet over the cheese.
6. Remove onto a plate. Garnish with parsley and serve.

Chicken and Vegetable Salad

 10 Minutes   0 minutes   2 servings   364 Kcal

INGREDIENTS

- 2 cups cooked chicken breast
- ½ cup carrots
- ½ cup finely chopped celery
- 1 cup chopped baby spinach
- 4 tbsp. non-fat sour cream
- 4 tsp. Dijon mustard
- 5 tbsp. fat-free mayonnaise
- 2 chopped tomatoes
- ½ cup low-fat shredded cheddar cheese
- Salt to taste
- Pepper to taste

PER SERVING

Proteins: 53.2 g
Carbohidrates: 15.3 g
Fat: 9.1 g

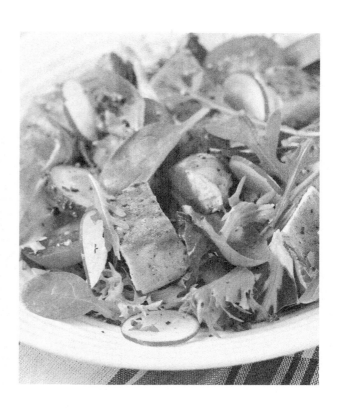

DIRECTIONS

1. Combine mustard, mayonnaise, cheese, and sour cream in a bowl.
2. Add chicken, carrots, tomatoes, celery, and spinach and incorporate well. Add salt and pepper to taste if desired.
3. Refrigerate until use. Eat chilled.

Bacon Pea Salad

 15 Minutes   0 minutes    3 servings   218 Kcal

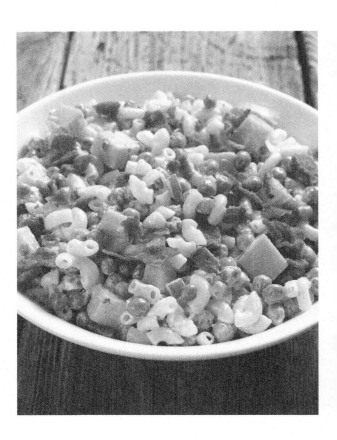

INGREDIENTS

- 2 cups frozen peas, thawed
- ¼ cup ranch salad dressing
- Salt to taste
- 2 bacon strips, cooked, crumbled
- ¼ shredded sharp cheddar cheese
- 3 tbsp. chopped red onion
- Pepper to taste

PER SERVING

Proteins: 8.0 g
Carbohidrates: 14.8 g
Fat: 14.3 g

DIRECTIONS

1. Combine peas, ranch salad dressing, salt, cheese, red onion, and pepper in a bowl.
2. Chill until ready to serve. Add bacon and stir.
3. Divide into 3 plates and serve.

Tortellini Salad, Zucchini and Peas

 20 Minutes 20 minutes 2 servings 302 Kcal

DIRECTIONS

1. Follow the instructions to cook, which are typically listed on the back package of pasta, and cook pasta without adding salt and fat.
2. Drop the peas into the pot of pasta during the last 6 minutes of cooking.
3. Drain in a colander and let it cool for 10 minutes. Transfer the pasta and peas into a bowl.
4. Heat 1 teaspoon of oil into a skillet. Add garlic and cook until it gets fragrant. Turn off the heat.
5. Stir in zucchini and keep stirring for about 60 – 70 seconds until the zucchini turns slightly soft.
6. Transfer zucchini into the bowl of pasta. Toss well.
7. Make the dressing by whisking together the remaining oil, lemon juice, lemon zest, pepper, and salt.
8. Drizzle dressing over the salad. Toss well and serve.

Black Bean Soup

 45 Minutes   35 minutes   2 servings   331 Kcal

INGREDIENTS

- 1-½ tbsp. olive oil
- ½ tbsp. ground cumin
- 1 can (14.5 ounces can) black beans
- ½ small red onion, finely chopped
- ½ medium onion, chopped
- 1 large clove garlic, minced
- 1 cup vegetable or chicken broth
- Pepper to taste
- A handful of fresh cilantro, chopped, to garnish
- Salt to taste

PER SERVING

Proteins: 16 g
Carbohidrates: 41 g
Fat: 12 g

DIRECTIONS

1. Trickle oil into a saucepan and heat over medium heat. Add onion once the oil is hot.
2. Stir often until the onion is soft. Stir in garlic. Cook for a few seconds until fragrant.
3. Stir in cumin and cook for a few seconds. Spoon broth into the saucepan and scrape the bottom of the saucepan to remove any particles that may be stuck.
4. Stir in half the black beans, all the liquid from the can of black beans, salt, and pepper. Let it boil for a couple of minutes. Turn off heat and lay to the side on a hot pad.
5. Put the soup in an immersion blender or in a fruit blender and turn on until smooth.
6. Add remaining black beans and stir.
7. Heat the soup thoroughly.
8. Divide the soup into 2 soup bowls. Garnish with cilantro and you are ready to eat.

Chicken & White Bean Soup

 25 Minutes   18 minutes   3 servings 248 Kcal

INGREDIENTS

- 1 tsp. extra-virgin olive oil
- ½ tbsp. chopped fresh sage
- 1 cup water
- 1 pound roasted chicken
- 1 leek, cut into ¼ inch round slices
- 1 can (14 ounces can) low-sodium chicken broth
- Pepper to taste
- ½ can (from a 15 ounces can) cannellini beans, rinsed, drained
- Salt to taste

PER SERVING

Proteins: 35.1 g
Carbohidrates: 14.8 g
Fat: 5.8 g

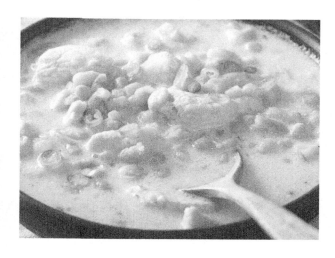

DIRECTIONS

1. Heat oil into a soup pot over medium-high flame. When oil is hot, add leeks and cook until they become slightly soft. Add sage and mix well. Cook for a few more seconds.
2. Add broth and water and stir. Cook covered on high heat.
3. Remove skin and bones from the chicken and cut or shred them into smaller pieces.
4. When the soup begins to boil, uncover and stir in chicken and beans. Heat thoroughly.
5. Divide the soup into 3 soup bowls. You can eat one and save the others for later meals or share with others.

Carrot and Lentil Soup

 25 Minutes   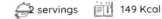 15 minutes   2 servings   149 Kcal

INGREDIENTS

- ½ tbsp. olive oil
- 1 medium carrot, peeled, finely chopped
- 2 cups vegetable stock
- A handful of fresh cilantro, chopped
- ½ small onion, chopped
- ⅛ cup red lentils
- Pepper to taste
- Chili flakes to taste
- Salt to taste

PER SERVING

Proteins: 7.7 g
Carbohidrates: 22.6 g
Fat: 3.6 g

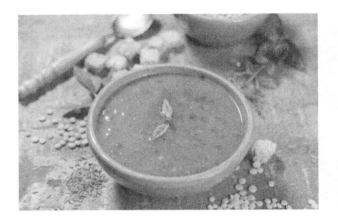

DIRECTIONS

1. Drizzle oil into a pan large enough for all ingredients and heat over medium heat. When oil is hot enough to start, add carrot and onion and sauté for a few minutes until onion turns translucent.
2. Add lentils and stir. Ladle stock and stir. Cook covered until the lentils and carrots are tender. Remove from the heat by setting it on the counter or a cool part of the stove.
3. Intermix the soup with an immersion blender or in a blender until smooth.
4. Add salt, pepper, and chili flakes to suit your taste and stir. Garnish with cilantro and serve.

Chicken and Chickpea Curry

45 Minutes 30 minutes 3 servings 309 Kcal

INGREDIENTS

- ¾ pound chicken breasts, diced
- 1½ tbsp. vegetable oil
- ½ onion, finely diced
- Salt to taste
- 2 cloves garlic, minced
- ½ tsp. turmeric powder
- 1 tbsp. yellow curry powder
- ¾ cup chicken stock
- 1 cup canned chickpeas, drained
- ½ cup drained, low-fat yogurt
- Pepper to taste

PER SERVING

Proteins: 3.5 g
Carbohidrates: 16.8 g
Fat: 2.1 g

DIRECTIONS

1. Take a heavy bottomed pan and heat oil over medium-high flame. When oil is hot, add the chicken and cook until brown.
2. Take out the chicken from the pan with a slotted spoon that will allow all juices to stay in the pan and place on a plate. Add garlic and onion into the pot and stir. Cook until soft.
3. Stir in turmeric powder and yellow curry powder.
4. Cook for about a minute or until you get a nice aroma taking care not to burn the spices.
5. Add chicken and mix with a spoon thoroughly. Add stock and stir. Cook covered for about 7 – 8 minutes.
6. Stir in yogurt and chickpeas and cook for another 5 – 7 minutes.
7. Serve over brown basmati rice or chapati.

Creamy Chicken & Mushrooms

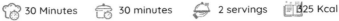 30 Minutes   30 minutes   2 servings   525 Kcal

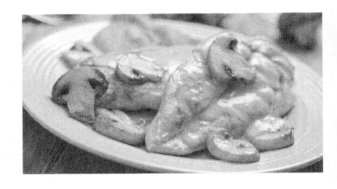

INGREDIENTS

- 2 chicken cutlets (4 - 5 ounces each)
- ¼ cup dry white wine
- 1 tbsp. finely chopped fresh parsley
- 2 cups mixed sliced mushrooms
- ¼ cup heavy cream
- Salt to taste
- Pepper to taste
- 1 tbsp. canola oil

PER SERVING

Proteins: 29.1 g
Carbohidrates: 4.2 g
Fat: 19.6 g

DIRECTIONS

1. Squirt ½ tablespoon oil into a skillet and heat over medium heat. Season the chicken and place it in the skillet.
2. Cook until the chicken is golden brown underneath. Turn the chicken over and cook the other side until brown and well-cooked inside. Remove chicken onto a plate.
3. Spoon ½ tablespoon oil into the pan. When oil is hot, add mushrooms and cook until tender.
4. Lower the heat and add cream and chicken along with cooking juices from the plate of chicken. Add salt and pepper to taste and stir.
5. Stir well. Divide into two plates. Garnish with parsley and it is ready to eat.

61

Grilled Salmon with Tomatoes

 35 Minutes   30 minutes   🍳 2 servings   📖 248 Kcal

INGREDIENTS

- 1 clove garlic, minced
- ½ tbsp. extra-virgin olive oil
- ¼ cup thinly sliced fresh basil leaves, divided
- Freshly ground pepper to taste
- ½ tsp. salt, divided
- ¾ pound wild salmon fillet
- 1 medium tomato, thinly sliced

PER SERVING

Proteins: 34.8 g
Carbohidrates: 3.1 g
Fat: 9.9 g

DIRECTIONS

1. Remove pin bones from the salmon, if any. Spray a large sheet of heavy-duty aluminum foil with some cooking spray and place the salmon over it with the skin side facing down.
2. To prepare your grill, whether outside or on the cabinet, turn it on to medium heat.
3. Place garlic and half the salt on your cutting board and mash with the back of a spoon until you get a paste.
4. Combine oil and the garlic paste in a bowl and spread it over the salmon. Scatter half the basil over the salmon and place tomato slices in an overlapping manner.
5. Sprinkle the remaining salt and some pepper on top. Lift the salmon along with foil and place it on the grill. Cook for about 10 – 12 minutes or until the fish flakes when you pierce with a fork.
6. Slide the salmon from the foil onto a plate. Cut the salmon into two equal pieces.
7. Garnish with remaining basil and best served warm.

Shrimp Oreganata Cauliflower Gnocchi

 20 Minutes 15 minutes 2 servings 133 Kcal

INGREDIENTS

- ½ bag (from a 12 ounces bag) frozen cauliflower gnocchi
- ½ tbsp. olive oil
- A large pinch dried oregano
- ½ pound cooked, peeled, shrimp (defrost if frozen)
- 1 cup halved grated potatoes
- 1 tsp. minced garlic
- Salt to taste

PER SERVING

Proteins: 2.2 g
Carbohidrates: 16.8 g
Fat: 5.5 g

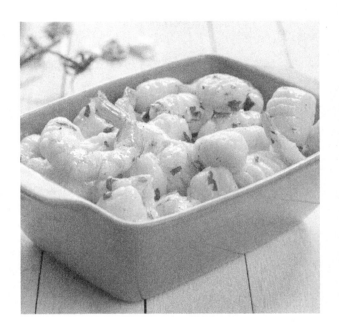

DIRECTIONS

1. Follow the directions on the package of cauliflower gnocchi and cook the gnocchi.
2. Place tomatoes, oregano, garlic, and salt in a microwave safe container. Drizzle oil on top and toss well.
3. Cook on High in the microwave for 50 – 60 seconds until slightly soft.
4. Add gnocchi and shrimp. Stir and you are ready for your meal.

Pork & Green Beans Stir-Fry

 15 Minutes   5 minutes   2 servings   387 Kcal

INGREDIENTS

- 2 tbsp. apricot jam
- ½ tbsp. toasted sesame oil
- ½ pound pork tenderloin, cut into thin strips
- 1-½ tbsp. avocado oil
- ⅛ cup thinly sliced scallions + extra to garnish
- 1 tbsp. soy sauce
- 1 tsp. chili-garlic sauce
- ⅛ cup cornstarch
- 6 oz. green beans, trimmed, cut into 2-inch pieces
- 1 tbsp. toasted sesame seeds

PER SERVING

Proteins: 27.6 g
Carbohidrates: 29,2 g
Fat: 19.0 g

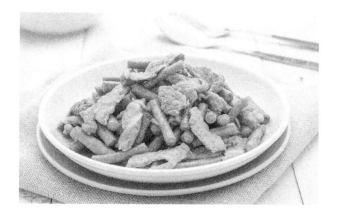

DIRECTIONS

1. Combine jam, sesame oil, tamari, and chili-garlic sauce in a bowl.
2. Place pork in a bowl and sprinkle cornstarch all over the pork.
3. Trickle grapeseed oil into a pan or cast-iron skillet and heat over medium–high heat.
4. When oil is hot, stir in the pork and cook until brown and crisp on both sides.
5. Add green beans and combine well. Cook until the beans are crisp as well as tender.
6. Spoon the jam mixture into the skillet and meld well. Turn off the heat.
7. Stir in scallions and sesame seeds. Garnish with extra scallions.

Beef and Beans

 30 Minutes   25 minutes   4 servings   185 Kcal

INGREDIENTS

- ¾ pound boneless round steak, cut into thin strips
- ½ tbsp. chili powder
- salt to taste
- 1 can (14.5 ounces) diced tomatoes
- ½ tsp. beef bouillon granules
- ½ tbsp. prepared mustard
- ½ can (16 ounces) kidney beans, rinsed, drained
- 2 small garlic cloves, minced
- ½ onion, chopped
- pepper to taste
- cooked brown rice

PER SERVING

Proteins: 24.2 g
Carbohidrates: 16.5 g
Fat: 3.1 g

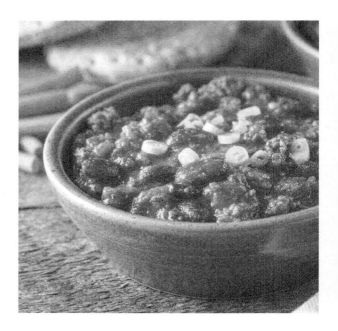

DIRECTIONS

1. Stir together mustard, salt, chili powder, garlic, and pepper in a bowl.
2. Transfer into a Dutch oven or slow cooker. Also add in the onion, tomatoes, and beef bouillon granules and stir. Cook covered until meat is cooked through.
3. Add beans and stir. Cook for a few more minutes and serve over any one of the suggested serving options.

Lamb & Fig Stew

 3 hours 3 hours 4 servings 📖 306 Kcal

INGREDIENTS

- 16 oz. lean ground lamb
- 4 tbsp. + 2 tbsp. minced garlic
- ½ cup dry red wine
- 4 tsp. cornstarch
- ½ cup dried figs, chopped
- Freshly ground pepper to taste
- 2 tsp. freshly grated lemon zest
- 2 tsp. extra-virgin olive oil
- 2 tsp. herbs de Provence
- 2 cans (14 oz.) beef broth
- 4 tomatoes, diced
- Salt to taste

PER SERVING

Proteins: 24.2 g
Carbohidrates: 23.8 g
Fat: 10.9 g

DIRECTIONS

1. Place a large saucepan, make sure all ingredients will fit in the pot over medium heat. Add lamb and stir. As you stir, break the meat as it cooks. Cook until meat turns brown, stirring often.
2. Remove lamb with a slotted spoon and position in a bowl to the side. Drain off the fat from the lamb.
3. Clean the pan. Sprinkle oil into the pan and heat over medium-high heat. When the oil is hot, add four tablespoons of garlic and herbs de Provence and sauté for a few seconds until fragrant. Stir constantly.
4. Add red wine and scrape the bottom to remove any burnt or browned bits that are stuck. Cook for 1 – 2 minutes.
5. Combine broth and cornstarch and add into the pan, stirring constantly.
6. Raise the heat to high heat. Stir in figs, tomatoes, and pepper. Lower the heat and allow to gently cook for 10-12 minutes.
7. Add lamb and salt and stir until well combined. Heat thoroughly and turn off the heat.
8. Ladle into bowls. Whisk together in a bowl, two teaspoons garlic, lemon zest, and sprinkle over the stew. Serve.

Black Bean Quesadillas

INGREDIENTS

- ½ can (15 oz.) black beans, drained, rinsed
- ¼ cup prepared fresh salsa, divided
- 1 tsp. canola oil, divided
- ¼ cup shredded Monterey Jack cheese
- 4 whole-wheat tortillas (8 inches each)
- ½ ripe avocado, peeled, pitted, diced

PER SERVING

Proteins: 13.2 g
Carbohidrates: 45.1 g
Fat: 16.3 g

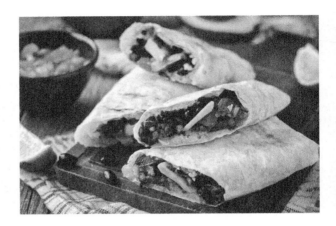

DIRECTIONS

1. Put together the beans, half the salsa, and cheese in a bowl. Divide the filling among the tortillas and spread it on one half of each of the tortillas.
2. Fold the plain or clean half of the tortilla over the filling.
3. Press slightly so that it is flat.
4. Heat a skillet over medium heat. Add ½ teaspoon oil and spread the oil in a skillet.
5. Place two quesadillas on the pan and cook until they turn s golden brown on both sides.
6. To serve: Place two quesadillas on each plate. Divide the avocado among the plates. Add a tablespoon of salsa on each plate.

Hearty Lentil and Brown Rice Burgers

 1 hour 20 minutes 6 servings 96 Kcal

INGREDIENTS

- 1 cup dried green lentils, rinsed
- 2 medium yellow onions, chopped
- 8 cloves garlic, minced
- 2 tsp. ground sage
- 3 cups water
- 1 cup brown rice
- 2 carrots, grated
- 6 tsp. ground cumin
- 2 tsp. sea salt or to taste
- 2 cups vegetable broth

PER SERVING

Proteins: 6.4 g
Carbohidrates: 21.5 g
Fat: 0.2 g

DIRECTIONS

1. Cook lentils, onion, cumin, salt, brown rice, carrot, sage, water, broth, and garlic in a saucepan and cook over medium heat. When the mixture comes to a boil, reduce the heat and cook until tender. If you have an instant pot or pressure cooker, you can prepare the lentil mixture in it. It will be much quicker. Transfer the lentil mixture into a colander. Let it sit for 3-4 minutes in the colander.
2. Transfer the lentil mixture into the food processor bowl and process until most of the lentils are nearly smooth.
3. Divide the mixture into six equal portions and shape it into patties. Spray some cooking spray over the patties.
4. You can cook the burgers on a preheated grill over medium heat for 5 minutes on each side or bake in a preheated oven at 350° F for roughly 25-30 minutes, or the tops look brown.
5. Serve over whole-wheat buns or over lettuce leaves with toppings of your choice.

Caprese Grilled Cheese

 10 Minutes   5 minutes   2 servings   272 Kcal

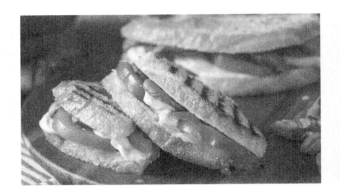

INGREDIENTS

- ½ cup shredded smoked mozzarella cheese
- 2 large slices whole-wheat country bread, halved or use 4 small slices
- 4 thin tomato slices
- 1-½ tbsp. pesto
- 1 tbsp. extra-virgin olive oil

PER SERVING

Proteins: 10.5 g
Carbohidrates: 14.4 g
Fat: 19.1 g

DIRECTIONS

1. Join together pesto and cheese and spread over two slices of the bread pieces.
2. Complete the sandwiches by topping with the remaining bread slices. Cover the sandwiches. Chill for a couple of hours. Unwrap and place two tomato slices in between each sandwich.
3. Brush oil on either side of the sandwiches and wrap each in heavy-duty foil.
4. Grill the sandwiches on a preheated grill until the sandwiches are crisp. Press occasionally with a spatula.
5. Unwrap carefully and slide onto serving plates.
6. It is advised to eat immediately.

Crispy Chickpeas

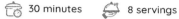 50 Minutes   30 minutes   8 servings   132 Kcal

INGREDIENTS

- 2 cans (15 ounces each) chickpeas, rinsed, drained.
- ½ tsp. smoked paprika
- 4 tsp. ground cumin
- ½ tsp. ground allspice
- 2 tsp. dried marjoram
- 2 tbsp. olive oil
- ½ tsp. salt or to taste
- ½ tsp. crushed red pepper
- 8 lime wedges to serve

PER SERVING

Proteins: 4.7 g
Carbohidrates: 14.1 g
Fat: 5.8 g

DIRECTIONS

1. Adjust the temperature of your oven to 250°F and heat up the oven.
2. Add oil and chickpeas into a bowl and toss well. Sprinkle salt, marjoram, and all the spices over the chickpeas and toss well. Spread the chickpeas onto a rimmed baking sheet.
3. Bake for about 25-30 minutes or until crisp. Stir the chickpeas every 8 – 10 minutes, spreading each time.
4. Remove chickpeas from the oven and transfer on to a plate lined with paper towels. Cool completely and store in an airtight container.
5. To serve: Place ¼ cup chickpeas in a bowl. Squeeze juice from the lemon wedge over the chickpeas. Toss well with forks or salad tongs.

Stuffed Mini Peppers

 10 Minutes 2 minutes 16 servings 15 Kcal

INGREDIENTS

- ½ tsp. cumin seeds
- ⅛ cup chopped fresh cilantro leaves + extra to garnish
- 1–½ tbsp. cider vinegar
- 8 miniature sweet pepper, halved lengthwise, deseeded
- ½ can (15 oz.) chickpeas, rinsed, drained
- 1–½ tbsp. water
- Salt to taste

PER SERVING

Proteins: 1.1 g
Carbohidrates: 3.7 g
Fat: 0.7 g

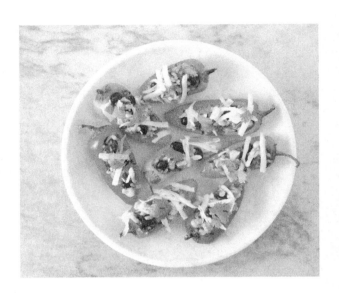

DIRECTIONS

1. Roast the cumin seeds in a small skillet placed over medium-low heat until you get a nice fragrance and slightly brown. Turn off the heat.
2. Blend together with a spoon the chickpeas, water, salt, cumin, cilantro, and cider vinegar in the food processor until well combined and smooth.
3. Fill this mixture into the pepper halves and place it on a plate. Sprinkle cilantro on top. Chill until use.

Mediterranean Pork Chops

 45 Minutes   10 minutes   2 servings   161 Kcal

INGREDIENTS

- 2 boneless or bone-in pork loin chops, about ½ inch thick
- Freshly ground pepper to taste
- 2 cloves garlic, minced
- Salt to taste
- ½ tbsp. finely snipped fresh rosemary or 1 tsp. dried rosemary, crushed

PER SERVING

Proteins: 24.9 g
Carbohidrates: 1.1 g
Fat: 5.8 g

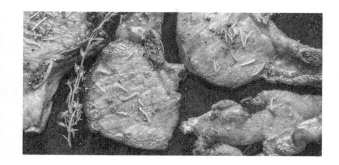

DIRECTIONS

1. Turn on the temperature of your oven to 425°F and preheat the oven. Prepare a roasting pan by lining it with aluminum foil. Place a rack in the roasting pan.
2. Season pork chops with salt and pepper. Make sure you season it all over.
3. Stir together rosemary and garlic in a bowl and scatter it all over the pork chops. Rub it well into the chops.
4. Place chops on the rack. Place the roasting pan along with the chops in the oven and roast for 10 minutes.
5. Now lower the temperature of the oven to 350°F and roast until the meat is not pink anymore. The internal temperature of the cooked meat should be 160°F when checked with a meat thermometer.

Pumpkin Pie in a Cup

 10 Minutes   0 minutes   2 servings   92 Kcal

INGREDIENTS

- 1 cup fat-free milk
- 6 tbsp. pure pumpkin puree
- 2 tbsp. thawed, low-fat frozen whipped topping
- ½ box (from a 1-ounce box) fat-free, sugar-free, instant vanilla pudding
- ½ tsp. pumpkin pie spice

PER SERVING

Proteins: 5.3 g
Carbohidrates: 16.8 g
Fat: 1.2 g

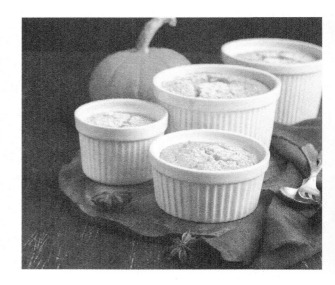

DIRECTIONS

1. Combine milk and vanilla pudding, blend in a bowl and stir with a spoon constantly until thick.
2. Add pumpkin puree and ¼ teaspoon pumpkin pie spice and whisk until well combined.
3. Divide the mixture into two pudding cups. Place the cups in the refrigerator for at least 2 – 3 hours or until use.
4. To serve: Place a tablespoon of whipped topping on top of each pudding. Garnish with remaining pumpkin pie spice.

Pineapple and Strawberry Paletas

 5 Minutes   0 minutes   4 servings   📖 31 Kcal

INGREDIENTS

- ¾ cup diced fresh pineapple
- ¾ cup diced fresh strawberries
- 3 tbsp. water
- Powdered stevia to taste or use any other artificial sweetener of your choice
- ½ tbsp. fresh lime juice

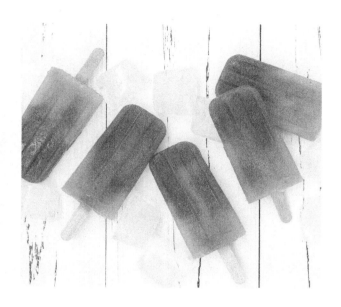

PER SERVING

Proteins: 0.8 g
Carbohidrates: 7.2 g
Fat: 0.7 g

DIRECTIONS

1. Place ½ tablespoon each of pineapple and strawberries into each of 4 Popsicle molds.
2. Place water, stevia, lime juice, and remaining pineapple and strawberries in a mixer and meld until smooth.
3. Spoon into the Popsicle molds and place the Popsicle sticks in it. Freeze until firm.
4. To serve, you can gently lower the Popsicle molds into a bowl of lukewarm water for 10 – 15 seconds. It will easily come off the mold.

1 - Week Meal Plan

Here is a sample meal plan you can follow to ensure you are consuming healthy and wholesome meals and snacks. For instance, if you are following the 16/8 method, you can have your first meal at noon, followed by a healthy snack in the evening, and a filling dinner at night. Alternatively, you can start your day with a hearty breakfast at 10 AM, have a light lunch at 1 PM, a smoothie at around 4 PM, and dinner at 6 PM. It is entirely up to you. Add 6 ounces of raw or cooked vegetables and one or two fresh fruits to at least one meal every day.

DAY	MEALS
1 - SUNDAY	Turkey sausage frittata
	Tortellini salad with zucchini and peas
	Sweet and sour chicken
2 - MONDAY	Goat cheese and ham omelet
	Chicken and vegetable salad
	Shrimp oreganata cauliflower gnocchi
3 - TUESDAY	Tomato cheddar cheese toast
	Bacon pea salad
	Grilled salmon with tomatoes and basil
4 - WEDNESDAY	Matcha smoothie
	Chicken and chickpea curry
	Carrot and lentil soup
5 - THURSDAY	Caprese grilled cheese
	Beef and beans
	Pork and green beans stir-fry
6 - FRIDAY	Strawberry avocado smoothie
	Creamy chicken and mushrooms
	Mediterranean pork chops
7 - SATURDAY	Matcha smoothie
	Chicken and white bean soup
	Hearty lentil and brown rice burgers

First Month of Intermittent Fasting

Well, shifting to intermittent fasting will change your life for the better. It's not just your physical health; your mental health will improve. Apart from this, you will feel stronger and energetic than ever before. That said, making a dietary change is not always easy. Learning about what to expect and mistakes to avoid, along with the tips to stay motivated, will ensure you stay on the right track. Following the simple suggestions and advice given in this chapter will improve the overall benefits associated with intermittent fasting.

It Takes Time

Do not think of intermittent fasting as a quick fix. Following this diet and getting used to it are two different things. It will take your body a couple of weeks to get accustomed to the eating and fasting protocols prescribed by intermittent fasting. Initially, prepare yourself for a little struggle. Once again, this depends on your usual diet and eating pattern. If you are not used to eating unhealthy foods or constantly snacking, shifting to any form of intermittent fasting protocol becomes easier. So, give you a body and mind a couple of weeks to get used to intermittent fasting.

Weight Loss

If you carefully follow the protocols of intermittent fasting and consume healthy and wholesome meals during the time frame allowed for eating, you will experience weight loss benefits. Even if it isn't much, you will lose a couple of pounds within a month. Because though the eating window or duration is fixed and has reduced significantly, your calorie consumption automatically reduces. Also, most of the weight loss during the initial weeks is associated with excess water stored within. When your body starts eliminating excess water, you start feeling less bloated. This is one benefit of intermittent fasting that leaves you feeling pleasantly surprised.

More Energy

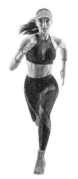

A wonderful thing about intermittent fasting is it increases and stabilizes your energy levels. Whenever you consume any foods rich in carbs or sugars, they are automatically converted into glucose. This causes a temporary spike in blood sugar levels. On the other hand, when your body is in a fasted state like it is on intermittent fasting, it starts utilizing internal fats or reserves for sustenance. These fat reserves will be

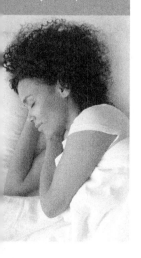

utilized until you eat foods that result in the production of glucose. Until then, your body is constantly producing energy. This is one of the reasons why your energy levels will stabilize while following intermittent fasting.

Even though intermittent fasting does not prescribe any restrictive food lists, by eating healthy and wholesome meals, you can improve your overall health. By opting for nutrient-dense foods, lean proteins, and dietary fibers, your body's nutritional requirements are automatically fulfilled. When you give your body the nutrients it needs for every life; it pays you back by functioning effectively and also improves. This will elevate your energy levels. This, coupled with a little exercise daily, will further enhance your energy levels.

Maintaining a Social Life

You don't have to compromise on your social life for the sake of a diet. This is one benefit of intermittent fasting that sets it apart when compared to all other diets. As long as you stick to the fasting and eating window prescribed by intermittent fasting, you don't have to think about anything else. Since this is the only rule, ensure that you follow it. So, all you need to do is simply schedule your social commitments such that it does not clash with your fasting window. This is quite a simple adjustment. Also, it is a small price to pay for all the diverse benefits associated with intermittent fasting.

Enjoying a Routine

An important aspect of intermittent fasting is it creates a schedule and structures your days. You can no longer eat whatever you please. Instead, you must follow the eating and fasting schedule prescribed by your chosen method of intermittent fasting. A well-structured day is synonymous with productivity too. When you have a proper schedule in place, making time for things that matter the most becomes easier. It also gives you better control over the food you eat.

Let's assume that you are following the 16/8 protocol of intermittent fasting. This means you need to fast for 16 hours while the eating window extends for 8-hours. Within this timeframe, you will need evenly spaced-out meals and snacks. To ensure that you consume healthy and wholesome meals, you will need to start cooking at home. To do this, a little meal prep is needed, along with grocery shopping. All the different recipes given in this book, along with the sample meal plan, will come in handy now. Feel free to create a meal plan that suits your tastes and preferences. When you know you are not allowed to eat beyond a specific time, you need to structure your day according to it. This means you will start eating, sleeping, and waking up consistently every single day. By adding a little exercise to your daily routine, your daily schedule becomes even better. When you start doing this, your body gets used to the schedule.

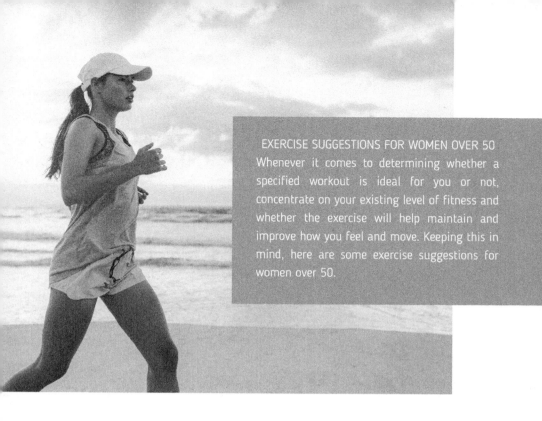

Brisk Walking

EXERCISE IS CRUCIAL REGARDLESS OF YOUR AGE

It's also vital for preserving your overall health and well-being. It's not restricted to physical well-being but includes your mental health too. Exercising will help you last longer and improve the quality of your life. Adding a little exercise to your daily routine will reduce the risk of several health problems, including heart diseases and low bone density.

One of the best workouts for your body is walking. Walking, especially after eating, can reduce and stabilize blood sugar levels by improving insulin functioning. Also, it's a pleasant way to work out. Going for a walk with your friend, listening to a podcast while walking, or even taking in the sights and sounds of nature can act as a stressbuster. If you can manage it, brisk walking is any day better than regular walking. By simply increasing the intensity of your walk, you can make most of the benefits it offers. According to the research undertaken by Zaccardi et al. (2018), brisk walking is associated with longer life expectancy.

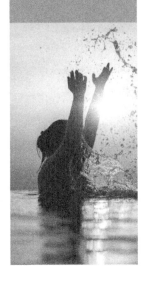

Weight-Bearing Exercises

As you age, the bone density starts reducing. By opting for resistance exercises, you can improve skeletal mass while reducing the load on bones. It also promotes the production of bone-forming cells and can help maintain bone mineral density in postmenopausal women, according to the findings of A Ram Hong and Sang Wan Kim (2018). Any weight-bearing exercise such as hiking, dancing, and even playing sports will do the trick. Resistance exercises such as lifting weights also strengthen the bones. Before you start engaging in any weight-bearing exercises, consult a professional and your healthcare provider.

Resistance Training

Loss of muscle mass and weakness are common as you age. Exercising to maintain muscle mass while staying functional and mobile is important. The simplest way to do this is by picking up weights, but what if this doesn't work for you? In such instances, opt for resistance training. It is a great way to challenge and strengthen your muscles, according to (Beckwee et al. 2019). A simple resistance exercise that supports your ability to pick things up like a deadlift. Instead, doing push-ups or even modified push-ups based on this ability will help you push. Any functional movement that mimics how your body moves daily is the best way to go about resistance training.

If you fast all day long and end the fast by snacking on unhealthy junk and processed foods, all your efforts go to waste. After all, what is the point of eating ice cream and chips for dinner after fasting for 16-hours? Even though there are no dietary rules in intermittent fasting, it's important to consume a well-balanced diet.

Biking

Physical activity combined with being outdoors can improve your cognitive health. According to a study undertaken by Leyland et al. (2019), biking regularly can improve your overall health executive functioning. If you don't like the idea of traditional biking, you can try an e-bike. There are stationary bikes as well.

Yoga

Yoga is not just restricted to touching your toes without bending your knees. There is so much more to it than performing complicated poses. You don't need extreme flexibility to perform yoga. That said, you can certainly build your strength, physical balance as well as flexibility with yoga. It's also a great way to improve your mental health and sleep

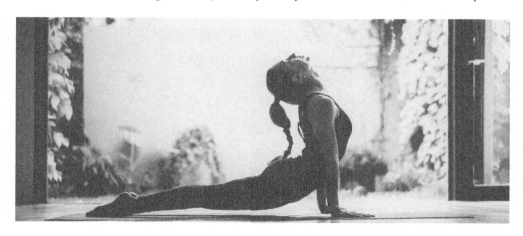

patterns, according to the findings of (Sivaramakrishnan et al. 2019). Apart from this, another benefit of yoga is that it is one activity that's ideal for women of all age groups, according to (Tulloch et al. 2018).

TIPS TO STAY MOTIVATED

Motivation refers to the internal urge that keeps you going despite any obstacles, setbacks, or hiccups you face. Motivation is needed in all aspects of life, and making dietary changes is not an exception. This is a primary difference between those who are successful and the ones who are still struggling. If you want to be the former, it's important to ensure your motivation level stays high while following intermittent fasting. Once you get into the groove, you will see positive results, which will increase your motivation to keep going. So here are some simple suggestions that will come in handy to stay motivated while making any dietary change.

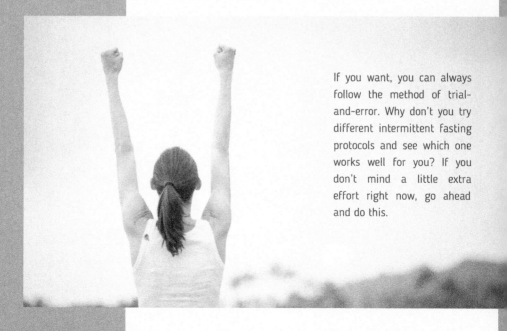

If you want, you can always follow the method of trial-and-error. Why don't you try different intermittent fasting protocols and see which one works well for you? If you don't mind a little extra effort right now, go ahead and do this.

Now that you have a list of goals that are motivating you to follow the diet, it's important to make a list of short-term goals as well. Establishing short-term goals helps improve your motivation levels. For instance, whenever you achieve a specific goal, it makes you feel better about yourself and increases your confidence to stick with your plan. By achieving multiple short-term goals, you are automatically closer to the long-term objective. So, any long-term goal established for intermittent fasting can be broken down into short-term goals.

Start by Making a List of Your Goals

Before you start following any protocol of intermittent fasting, it's important to make a list of your goals. Goals give you direction and purpose. They also ensure you are on the right track. You need to establish goals in your personal as well as professional lives. Take some time, and think about all the different reasons that prompt you to make the dietary changes prescribed by intermittent fasting. The goals can be small or big. As long as the goal matters to you and holds some personal value, it will be a motivating factor. For instance, a goal can be weight loss and maintenance or increasing your energy levels. Whatever your goal is, make a note of it. Your goals don't have to be the same numbers.

Whenever you are establishing goals, ensure that they are measurable, attainable, relevant, and time-bound. If the goal doesn't include any of these conditions, the chances of succeeding reduce automatically. To avoid this, it's important to ensure your goals are not vague and are quite descriptive. If weight loss is your priority, your goal cannot be, "I want to lose weight," or "I need to drop all these extra pounds." The goal is quite vague and doesn't tell you what you are supposed to do, how to do it, or when to do it. Instead of this, here is an example of a good goal- "I want to lose 20 lbs within six months by following intermittent fasting." This goal is not only attainable but comes with a time limit making it more realistic.

You can turn the goals you have created in the previous steps into positive affirmations. Simply repeat your goals out loud for five minutes daily. Say them out loud, repeat them in your mind, or write them down.

Feed Your Mind

A simple yet effective means to improve your motivation levels is by becoming mindful of the content you feed your mind. The human mind is an incredibly powerful tool. Unfortunately, most don't realize that their mind is under their control, and it shouldn't be the other way around. Now, it's time to start filtering the content you feed your mind to ensure it gets only motivating or inspiring information. If you are constantly feeding your brain

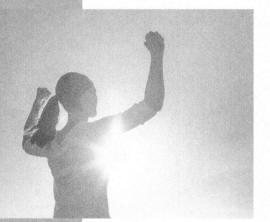

negative information from internal and external sources, it will get accustomed to a negative thinking pattern. To break free of this pattern, you need to become mindful of feeding it positive information. Making a dietary change is not easy, especially if you have not followed any specific eating protocols in the last couple of decades. Now that you are making a significant dietary change in your 50s, it's important to understand the journey will not be easy. There will be hurdles, and there will be thoughts that can quickly derail or prevent you from sticking to the schedule. On such days, it's important to understand you are alone. Reach out to your support system or even a support group online. Spend time with others who are facing similar struggles.

CARROT AND STICK
APPROACH
You might have
heard of the carrot
and stick approach.
The analogy it is
based on is that a
stick or a carrot can
be used for
motivating the
donkey to move
along. It means you
can motivate
yourself using
punishment or a
reward. It depends
on you what seems
to be motivating to
you. For instance,
you can treat
yourself to
something you've
been meaning to buy
if you achieve one of
your goals. On the
other hand, a
punishment for not
achieving the same
could be abstaining
from eating your
favorite food for a
month. Or maybe
increasing the time
spent exercising. By
simply thinking
about things that
you have no interest
or inclination to do,
it increases your
motivation to do
what you are
supposed to do.

Create Accountability

Humans have a basic tendency to follow through on promises or commitments they share with others. When you share an idea, goal, or aspiration with others, you automatically feel accountable to them. You can use this tendency to increase your motivation while following a diet. In the previous chapter, it was said that you need a support system in place before starting a diet. Now, it's time to start creating some accountability. Share the goals you have established so far with your support system. Ask them to check in on you and keep track of the progress you are making. When you do this, the external pressure to achieve the goals and prove yourself right will be higher. This itself acts as a motivating factor. On those days when you don't want to follow the intermittent fasting protocols, exercise, or do anything else recommended by this diet, simply remind yourself of the commitment you made.

Concentrate on the positive

Another simple way to motivate yourself is by concentrating on all the benefits associated with attaining the goals you have set. Apart from this, think about the different benefits associated with intermittent fasting you were introduced to in the previous chapter. Make a note of everything you stand to gain by making the dietary change. When in doubt, or whenever your motivation levels drop, simply remind yourself of everything you will gain.

Check Progress

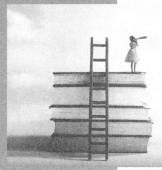

At times, it might feel as if you cannot even see the finishing line. When this happens, your motivation levels to keep going automatically reduce. In such instances, instead of getting worried looking at the distance you have to cover, look at how far you have come. Even within a few weeks of following this diet, you will see some positive changes in your body. Some changes are noticeable, while others can not be felt.

For instance, you will feel more energetic. On the other hand, you might notice a reduction in your body measurements even if the scales stay the same. So, it's important to make a note of all your non-scalable victories and not just the scalable ones. Before the diet starts, take some time and make a note of your body measurements. Similarly, take a picture of yourself and keep it as a motivation. Now after a couple of weeks, check your measurements, and you might notice a change. If they have reduced, it means the diet is working. Similarly, if any of your older clothes fit you better, it's also a sign that diet is working!

VISUALIZATION

You can also use a simple technique known as visualization to increase your motivation levels to keep going. Remember, in the previous point; it was said that you need to concentrate on the positive aspects of a specific topic to increase your motivation to keep going. Similarly, by visualizing a future your desire or imagining how you will feel after achieving your goals, you are creating a positive visualization. Make this visualization as clear and detailed as you can. Concentrate on all the small details.

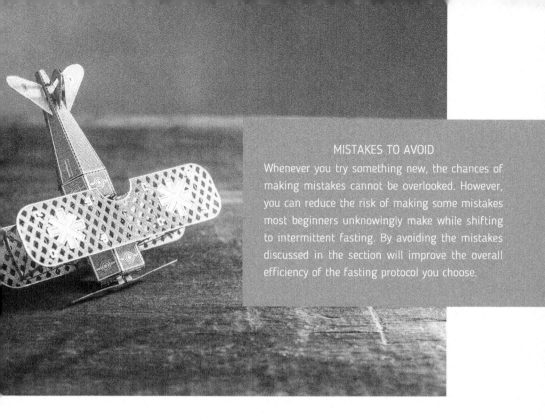

MISTAKES TO AVOID
Whenever you try something new, the chances of making mistakes cannot be overlooked. However, you can reduce the risk of making some mistakes most beginners unknowingly make while shifting to intermittent fasting. By avoiding the mistakes discussed in the section will improve the overall efficiency of the fasting protocol you choose.

NOT EXERCISING REGULARLY

If you are genuinely mesmerized in improving your well-being and health, exercising regularly must be the norm, not an exception. Add at least 30 minutes of exercise to your daily routine. You don't have to spend hours together, and you don't have to engage in any activity you don't want to. Try to find any activity that gets your body moving and stick with it consistently.

Selecting the Wrong Intermittent Fasting Plan

Another common mistake you need to avoid is selecting the wrong intermittent fasting protocol. Certain intermittent fasting protocols might work for some, while they are not ideal for others. So, it is important to ensure that you pick up a protocol that works for you. Don't just go with something because it seems to be working for others. For instance, if you are used to skipping breakfast regularly, following the 16/8 method is ideal. Similarly, if the intermittent fasting protocol you opt for is clashing with your social life, following it, in the long run, becomes quite difficult. As mentioned, for the diet to be sustainable, it needs to work with your lifestyle and not against it.

Consuming Wrong Foods During the Eating Window

Intermittent fasting does not have any strict protocols about the food you can and cannot eat. That said, be a little prudent if you want to improve your overall health and well-being. Suppose you start filling up on refined sugars, carbs, or fatty foods, the chances of overheating increase. Apart from that, feeding your body nutrient-devoid foods rich in calories will only increase your calorie consumption without giving your body its required nutrients.

Instead, you need to opt for healthy and wholesome ingredients such as unrefined grains, greens, healthy fats, lean protein, nuts, and wholesome vegetables. Whenever you are purchasing any food items, carefully read through the list of ingredients on the nutritional labels. If there are any items on it you cannot recognize or understand, avoid such products altogether. It's not just about consuming the wrong ingredients; eating too much during the eating window is undesirable too. Just because you are not going to be consuming any food during the fasting window doesn't mean you need to overcompensate during the eating window. As a rule of thumb, eat only until you are full. Once you feel full, stop eating. It is okay even if you cannot finish the required portions you have set aside for the eating window. When you start paying attention to when you feel full and hungry, your ability to regulate your appetite also improves.

Severe Calorie Restriction During the Eating Window

A calorie deficit is needed for weight loss. That said, if you severely restrict your calorie consumption, it will do your body more harm than good. Yes, there is such a thing as eating too little. Remember the food you consume during the eating window acts as sustenance through the fasting window. If you consume less than 1200 calories daily, it shifts your body into starvation mode. Once this happens, it stops burning calories and instead starts hoarding them. It can also sabotage your metabolic rate resulting in loss of muscle mass.

Not Keeping Your Body Hydrated

The importance of keeping your body hydrated cannot be overstressed. If you are just getting started with intermittent fasting, chances are you might experience muscle cramps, intense hunger pangs, or even headaches. Most of these symptoms are associated with dehydration. So, keep your body thoroughly hydrated. Apart from water, you can also consume some apple cider vinegar to curb hunger pangs, unsweetened black coffee, and unsweetened green, black, or herbal teas. When it comes to hydration, it's not just about drinking sufficient water. You must pay attention to your electrolyte levels as well. For instance, if you drink multiple cups of coffee or tea, most of the electrolytes present within are removed. You need to replace these electrolytes, or you will be dehydrated. Glauber's salts, baking soda, and apple cider vinegar will come in handy.

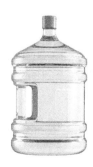

Not Forgiving Yourself

We are all human and, therefore, are bound to make mistakes at one point or another. Making mistakes is not a problem. How you deal with them is all that matters. If you let a mistake define you and your life, you cannot get anything done or get anywhere. On the other hand, if you think of a mistake as a learning opportunity, learn your lessons, move on, the

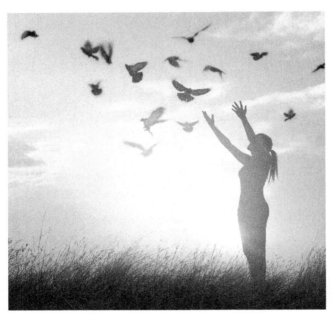

chances of repeating the mistake are reduced. There will be days when you might not be able to complete the fast first of days when you don't want to fast altogether. Maybe there are days when you want to eat something you're not supposed to. On all such days, be a little compassionate. Little self-compassion goes a long way in maintaining the required motivation to keep going. If you treat a mistake as a failure or the end of the road, it will become a self-fulfilling prophecy. Think of it as a simple setback, learn from it, and avoid repeating the same mistake in the future.

AVOID SOLID FOOD
as a rule of thumb. That said, if you are unable to make it through the fasting window, it's okay. Cut yourself some slack and try again. If the fasting window is too long, customize it. There is no reason why you shouldn't customize intermittent fasting protocols according to your convenience. As long as you are consuming healthy and wholesome meals and you exercising regularly, your health will improve.

Unknowingly Breaking Fast

A common mistake most beginners make is they are unknowingly breaking their fast. This usually happens when you consume hidden calories. For instance, fruit juices might seem healthy, but they are all not the same. Freshly squeezed fruit juice is healthier than the packaged ones. That said, drinking fruit juice during a 16/8 fast is not a good idea because the calories present in it will throw your body out of ketosis. Consuming any beverage or food that includes calories will shift your body from a fast to a fed state. The simplest way to avoid this is by sticking to the beverage suggestions discussed in the previous chapters.

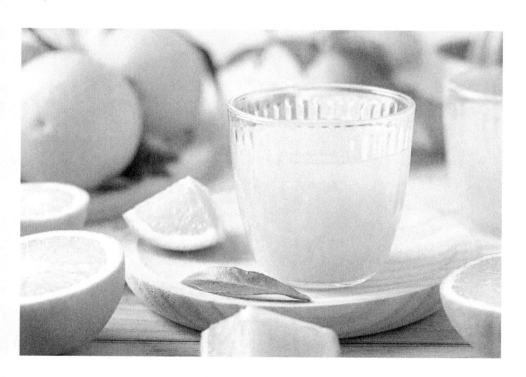

HEALTHY DIET
TIPS AND SUGGESTIONS

Apart from all the different types and suggestions mentioned until now, here are some additional tips you can use to improve your overall health and ensure that you are following a healthy eating pattern.

Start Your Day with Water

How you start your day matters a lot. The first thing you do and how you feel in the morning sets the path for the rest of the day. If you start on a good note, you will automatically feel better about yourself all day long. A healthy practice is to begin your day with a glass of water. Drinking about 250 ml of water first

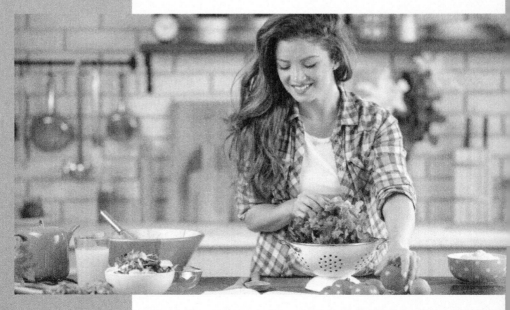

thing in the morning is believed to improve your metabolism and aid in better digestion. Add half a lemon to it, and it will further improve your digestive system. This is better than starting your day with fruit juices that might contain hidden carbs and calories that your body doesn't need.

Reduce Sugar Consumption

Consumption of sugar, especially refined sugars found in most prepackaged and processed food, is incredibly harmful. Excess sugar consumption is associated with an increased risk of diabetes, cardiovascular disorders, and even strokes. Apart from this, it also wreaks havoc on your digestive health. Avoid all this and reduce your sugar consumption. In fact, instead of white and processed sugar, opt for natural sweeteners such as dates, honey, maple syrup, stevia, and agave.

Increase Calcium Intake

Bone density along with physical strength reduces as women go through menopause. This is an inevitable change, but there are certain tips you can do to ensure it doesn't become a significant problem. The simplest way to ensure this doesn't happen is by increasing your calcium intake. From using a supplement to consuming calcium-fortified foods and beverages, you can keep brittle bones away. Consult your healthcare provider to determine the ideal daily dose of calcium.

Avoid Oily Foods

Oily foods are associated with an increased risk of high levels of cholesterol. Apart from this, they also increase the risk of atherosclerosis and plaque build-up within the arteries. A combination of all these factors is associated with poor cardiovascular help. As with sugars, even oily foods there are rich in trans fats, and hydrogenated oils harm your digestive health. Avoid fried foods as much as you possibly can. Whether they are French fries, chips, or even chicken wings, avoid fried foods and instead replace them with healthier options. For instance, baked kale chips, baked sweet potato fries, or even air-fried chicken wings are healthier selections. All it takes is a little thought and creativity so you can eat your favorite food without the added guilt.

Preventive Screenings

To stay on top of your health means you should know how healthy you are right now. Mammograms, heart scans, lung scans, other types of body scans, and even regular blood tests are all preventive screening measures. If there are any potential problems, these diagnostic tools help detect the problem even before it escalates or manifests. The risk of certain disorders increases as you age. Preventive screenings ensure you are one step ahead of your health and are living the best life possible.

Pay Attention to Sodium Intake

To improve your heart health, you need to cut back on salt. Pay extra attention to your sodium intake after reaching the big five-oh! Excess sodium harms your body in different ways. From increasing the risk of stroke and kidney diseases to heart attacks and high blood pressure, these are all preventable conditions. Frozen food, canned food, fast food, and salty snacks are all filled with sodium that your body does not need. By avoiding most processed foods, you can easily regulate your sodium and a. You can add more herbs and spices to flavor the food instead of relying on salt.

Strength Training Helps

Intermittent fasting doesn't increase the risk of muscle loss, provided you carefully follow the protocols it lays down. If you exercise too hard and don't eat enough, muscle loss occurs. That said, a little exercise helps reduce the risk of muscle loss. Add strength training to your daily routine for gaining and improving muscle mass while promoting weight loss and its maintenance. The benefits of exercise cannot be overlooked. Exercise refines your health, both physically and mentally. Whenever you exercise, plenty of feel-good hormones known as endorphins are released in your body. They help counteract the damaging effects of stress-related hormones such as cortisol.

The importance of sleep cannot be overstressed. Whenever you sleep, your body gets a break from its conscious activities and can focus on healing and repairing itself on the inside. It also starts utilizing the stored reserves when you are asleep. Sleep is rejuvenating and restorative. When you get a good night's rest, you automatically feel fresher, energetic, and motivated to get through your day. On the other hand, you'll feel down in the dumps, low on energy, and irritable when you don't get sufficient sleep. So, you must create and maintain a consistent sleep schedule to ensure your body gets at least seven hours of good quality undisturbed sleep at night. Sufficient sleep coupled with exercise and a healthy diet will automatically improve your overall health and well-being.

Keep Yourself Distracted During Fasts

Whenever you are fasting, ensure that your mind is thoroughly occupied or distracted. Have you ever noticed that you don't feel hungry or don't experience any food cravings when you are busy doing other things? This is because your mind is focused on other things to concentrate on anything. You might have also realized the urge to eat, especially unhealthy and junk food, increases when you are bored. So, keep yourself occupied during the fasting window to make things easier. Use this time to engage in any of your hobbies or learn a new skill if you want.

Maintain a Food Journal

Start maintaining the food journal to get a better insight into the food choices you are making. It is also a great way to become mindful of the calories you are consuming. Certain calories are helpful while others are harmful. Healthy calories include the ones obtained from healthy and wholesome food, while unhealthy calories are present in cabs, sugars, and processed foods. If you want to lose weight or fat and maintain the results, you need to become conscious of the food choices you make. You can always make a note of what you are consuming in a diary or even use an online application to do the same.

Conclusion

You might have heard that age is just a number. Well, it is! You don't have to let age get in the way of living and enjoying your life to the fullest. Regardless of whether you have just reached the big five-oh or past it, there is plenty in store for you. That's said, one thing that does not change is your responsibility toward keeping yourself healthy. Taking care of your health will always be your responsibility. Whether it's your mental or physical well-being, neither can be overlooked. Now, you need to take a little more care of your body to ensure it functions effectively and efficiently.

A great way to improve your overall health and fitness levels is by following the protocols of intermittent fasting. This is an incredibly genuine dietary protocol that switches it up between fasting and eating. Intermittent fasting is one of the simplest ways to improve your overall health. From achieving and maintaining your weight loss goals to improving your cardiovascular health, tackling insomnia, and improving your metabolism, and reducing the risk of different health problems, this diet is truly wonderful. Also, it is sustainable in the long run, unlike most crash and fad diets that promise big results and don't deliver. All the benefits offered by intermittent fasting are backed by science, and you can gain them all by following the simple advice, tips, and suggestions given in this book.

Don't forget to go through all the different healthy, simple, and delicious intermittent fasting-friendly recipes given in this book. By following this diet, you can improve your overall health without obsessing about every calorie consumed! Simply shift your focus to when you eat and follow the fasting window prescribed by your chosen method of intermittent fasting.

So, what are you waiting for? All the information you need about intermittent fasting and simple suggestions to get started with it were discussed in this book. Now, you simply need to get started with intermittent fasting. Yes, it actually is as simple as that. Once you get accustomed to intermittent fasting, you will notice a positive revamping in your well-being.

Thank you and all the best!

the Author

Emily Walker

References

Aksungar, F. B., Topkaya, A. E., & Akyildiz, M. (2007). Interleukin-6, C-reactive protein and biochemical parameters during prolonged intermittent fasting. Annals of Nutrition & Metabolism, 51(1), 88–95. https://doi.org/10.1159/000100954

Alirezaei, M., Kemball, C. C., Flynn, C. T., Wood, M. R., Whitton, J. L., & Kiosses, W. B. (2010). Short-term fasting induces profound neuronal autophagy. Autophagy, 6(6), 702–710. https://doi.org/10.4161/auto.6.6.12376

Arnason, T. G., Bowen, M. W., & Mansell, K. D. (2017). Effects of intermittent fasting on health markers in those with type 2 diabetes: A pilot study. World Journal of Diabetes, 8(4), 154. https://doi.org/10.4239/wjd.v8.i4.154

Baier, L. (2020, April 18). 9 Intermittent Fasting Mistakes (And How To Avoid Them!). A Sweet Pea Chef. https://www.asweetpeachef.com/intermittent-fasting-mistakes/

BaHammam, A., Almeneessier, A., Alzoghaibi, M., BaHammam, A., Ibrahim, M., Olaish, A., & Nashwan, S. (2018). The effects of diurnal intermittent fasting on the wake-promoting neurotransmitter orexin-A. Annals of Thoracic Medicine, 13(1), 48. https://doi.org/10.4103/atm.atm_181_17

Beckwée, D., Delaere, A., Aelbrecht, S., Baert, V., Beaudart, C., Bruyere, O., de Saint-Hubert, M., & Bautmans, I. (2019). Exercise Interventions for the Prevention and Treatment of Sarcopenia. A Systematic Umbrella Review. The Journal of Nutrition, Health & Aging, 23(6), 494–502. https://doi.org/10.1007/s12603-019-1196-8

Bhutani, S., Klempel, M. C., Kroeger, C. M., Trepanowski, J. F., & Varady, K. A. (2013). Alternate day fasting and endurance exercise combine to reduce body weight and favorably alter plasma lipids in obese humans. Obesity, 21(7), 1370–1379. https://doi.org/10.1002/oby.20353

Chiofalo, B., Laganà, A. S., Palmara, V., Granese, R., Corrado, G., Mancini, E., Vitale, S. G., Ban Frangež, H., Vrtačnik-Bokal, E., & Triolo, O. (2017). Fasting as a possible complementary approach for polycystic ovary syndrome: Hope or hype? Medical Hypotheses, 105, 1–3. https://doi.org/10.1016/j.mehy.2017.06.013

Dong, T. A., Sandesara, P. B., Dhindsa, D. S., Mehta, A., Arneson, L. C., Dollar, A. L., Taub, P. R., & Sperling, L. S. (2020). Intermittent Fasting: A Heart Healthy Dietary Pattern? The American Journal of Medicine, 133(8). https://doi.org/10.1016/j.amjmed.2020.03.030

Faris, M. A.-I. E., Kacimi, S., Al-Kurd, R. A., Fararjeh, M. A., Bustanji, Y. K., Mohammad, M. K., & Salem, M. L. (2012). Intermittent fasting during Ramadan attenuates proinflammatory cytokines and immune cells in healthy subjects. Nutrition Research, 32(12), 947–955. https://doi.org/10.1016/j.nutres.2012.06.021

Hartman, M. L., Veldhuis, J. D., Johnson, M. L., Lee, M. M., Alberti, K. G., Samojlik, E., & Thorner, M. O. (1992). Augmented growth hormone (GH) secretory burst frequency and amplitude mediate enhanced GH secretion during a two-day fast in normal men. The Journal of Clinical Endocrinology and Metabolism, 74(4), 757–765. https://doi.org/10.1210/jcem.74.4.1548337

Heilbronn, L., Smith, S., Martin, C., Anton, S., & Ravussin. (2005, January 1). Alternate-day Fasting in Nonobese Subjects: Effects on Body Weight, Body Composition, and Energy Metabolism. The American Journal of Clinical Nutrition. https://pubmed.ncbi.nlm.nih.gov/15640462/

Hong, A. R., & Kim, S. W. (2018). Effects of Resistance Exercise on Bone Health. Endocrinology and Metabolism, 33(4), 435. https://doi.org/10.3803/enm.2018.33.4.435

Ho, K. Y., Veldhuis, J. D., Johnson, M. L., Furlanetto, R., Evans, W. S., Alberti, K. G., & Thorner, M. O. (1988). Fasting enhances growth hormone secretion and amplifies the complex rhythms of growth hormone secretion in man. Journal of Clinical Investigation, 81(4), 968–975. https://www.ncbi.nlm.nih.gov/pmc/articles/PMC329619/

Lee, J., Herman, J. P., & Mattson, M. P. (2000). Dietary Restriction Selectively Decreases Glucocorticoid Receptor Expression in the Hippocampus and Cerebral Cortex of Rats. Experimental Neurology, 166(2), 435–441. https://doi.org/10.1006/exnr.2000.7512

Lee, C., Raffaghello, L., Brandhorst, S., Safdie, F. M., Bianchi, G., Martin-Montalvo, A., Pistoia, V., Wei, M., Hwang, S., Merlino, A., Emionite, L., de Cabo, R., & Longo, V. D. (2012). Fasting cycles retard growth of tumors and sensitize a range of cancer cell types to chemotherapy. Science Translational Medicine, 4(124), 124ra27. https://doi.org/10.1126/scitranslmed.3003293

Leyland, L.-A., Spencer, B., Beale, N., Jones, T., & van Reekum, C. M. (2019). The effect of cycling on cognitive function and well-being in older adults. PLOS ONE, 14(2), e0211779. https://doi.org/10.1371/journal.pone.0211779

Li, L., Wang, Z., & Zuo, Z. (2013). Chronic intermittent fasting improves cognitive functions and brain structures in mice. PloS One, 8(6), e66069. https://doi.org/10.1371/journal.pone.0066069

Martin, B., Mattson, M. P., & Maudsley, S. (2006). Caloric restriction and intermittent fasting: Two potential diets for successful brain aging. Ageing Research Reviews, 5(3), 332-353. https://doi.org/10.1016/j.arr.2006.04.002

Migala, J. (2021, May 3). 6 Best Exercises for Women Over 50. EatingWell. https://www.eatingwell.com/article/7900848/best-exercises-for-women-over-50/

Pierce, J. J. (2020, July 27). 8 Health Tips for Women Over 50. Preventative Diagnostic Center. https://www.pdcenterlv.com/blog/8-health-tips-for-women-over-50/

Rasmussen, M. H. (2010). Obesity, growth hormone and weight loss. Molecular and Cellular Endocrinology, 316(2), 147–153. https://doi.org/10.1016/j.mce.2009.08.017

Rasmussen, M. H., Hvidberg, A., Juul, A., Main, K. M., Gotfredsen, A., Skakkebaek, N. E., Hilsted, J., & Skakkebae, N. E. (1995). Massive weight loss restores 24-hour growth hormone release profiles and serum insulin-like growth factor-I levels in obese subjects. The Journal of Clinical Endocrinology & Metabolism, 80(4), 1407–1415. https://doi.org/10.1210/jcem.80.4.7536210

Rocha, N. S., Barbisan, L. F., de Oliveira, M. L. C., & de Camargo, J. L. V. (2002). Effects of fasting and intermittent fasting on rat hepatocarcinogenesis induced by diethylnitrosamine. Teratogenesis, Carcinogenesis, and Mutagenesis, 22(2), 129–138. https://doi.org/10.1002/tcm.10005

Roelfsema, F., Yang, R. J., & Veldhuis, J. D. (2018). Differential Effects of Estradiol and Progesterone on Cardiovascular Risk Factors in Postmenopausal Women. Journal of the Endocrine Society, 2(7), 794–805. https://doi.org/10.1210/js.2018-00073

Salgin, B., Marcovecchio, M., Hill, N., Dunger, D., & Frystyk, J. (2012, April 1). The Effect of Prolonged Fasting on Levels of Growth Hormone-Binding Protein and Free Growth Hormone. Growth Hormone & IGF Research : Official Journal of the Growth Hormone Research Society and the International IGF Research Society. https://pubmed.ncbi.nlm.nih.gov/22386777/

Sivaramakrishnan, D., Fitzsimons, C., Kelly, P., Ludwig, K., Mutrie, N., Saunders, D. H., & Baker, G. (2019). The effects of yoga ..... review and meta-analysis of randomised controlled trials. The International Journal of Behavioral Nutrition and Physical Activity, 16(1), 33. https://doi.org/10.1186/s12966-019-0789-2

Tajes, M., Gutierrez-Cuesta, J., Folch, J., Ortuño-Sahagun, D., Verdaguer, E., Jiménez, A., Junyent, F., Lau, A., Camins, A., & Pallàs, M. (2010). Neuroprotective role of intermittent fasting in senescence-accelerated mice P8 (SAMP8). Experimental Gerontology, 45(9), 702–710. https://doi.org/10.1016/j.exger.2010.04.010

Tinsley, G. M., & La Bounty, P. M. (2015). Effects of intermittent fasting on body composition and clinical health markers in humans. Nutrition Reviews, 73(10), 661–674. https://doi.org/10.1093/nutrit/nuv041

Tulloch, A., Bombell, H., Dean, C., & Tiedemann, A. (2018). Yoga-based exercise improves health-related quality of life and mental well-being in older people: a systematic review of randomised controlled trials. Age and Ageing, 47(4), 537–544. https://doi.org/10.1093/ageing/afy044

Varady, K. A., Bhutani, S., Church, E. C., & Klempel, M. C. (2009). Short-term modified alternate-day fasting: a novel dietary strategy for weight loss and cardioprotection in obese adults. The American Journal of Clinical Nutrition, 90(5), 1138–1143. https://doi.org/10.3945/ajcn.2009.28380

Zaccardi, F., Davies, M. J., Khunti, K., & Yates, T. (2019). Comparative Relevance of Physical Fitness and Adiposity on Life Expectancy: A UK Biobank Observational Study. Mayo Clinic Proceedings, 94(6), 985–994. https://doi.org/10.1016/j.mayocp.2018.10.029

Zauner, C., Schneeweiss, B., Kranz, A., Madl, C., Ratheiser, K., Kramer, L., Roth, E., Schneider, B., & Lenz, K. (2000). Resting energy expenditure in short-term starvation is increased as a result of an increase in serum norepinephrine. The American Journal of Clinical Nutrition, 71(6), 1511–1515. https://doi.org/10.1093/ajcn/71.6.1511

Zhao, D., Guallar, E., Ouyang, P., Subramanya, V., Vaidya, D., Ndumele, C. E., Lima, J. A., Allison, M. A., Shah, S. J., Bertoni, A. G., Budoff, M. J., Post, W. S., & Michos, E. D. (2018). Endogenous Sex Hormones and Incident Cardiovascular Disease in Post-Menopausal Women. Journal of the American College of Cardiology, 71(22), 2555–2566. https://doi.org/10.1016/j.jacc.2018.01.083

Temperature

F ° FAHRENHEIT	C° CELSIUS
100 °F	37 °C
150 °F	65 °C
200 °F	93 °C
250 °F	121 °C
300 °F	150 °F
325 °F	160 °C
350 °F	180 °C
375 °F	190 °C
400 °F	200 °C
425 °F	220 °C
450 °F	230°C
500 °F	260 °C
525 °F	274 °C
550 °F	288 °C

Volume

CUP	TBSP	TSP	ML.
1 C.	16 tbsp.	48 tsp.	237 ml.
3/4 C.	12 tbsp.	36 tsp.	177 ml.
2/3 C.	10.5 tbsp.	32 tsp.	158 ml.
1/2 C.	8 tbsp.	24 tsp.	118 ml.
1/3 C.	5.5 tbsp.	16 tsp.	79 ml.
1/4 C.	4 tbsp.	12 tsp.	59 ml.
1/6 C.	2.5 tbsp.	8 tsp.	40 ml.
1/8 C.	2 tbsp.	6 tsp.	30 ml.
1/16 C.	1 tbsp.	3 tsp.	15 ml.

Weight

IMPERIAL	METRIC
1 ounce	29 g.
2 oz.	57 g.
3 oz.	85 g.
4 oz.	113 g.
5 oz.	141 g.
6 oz.	170 g.
7 oz.	202 g.
8 oz.	227 g.
1 pound	435 g.
2 lb.	870 g.
3 lb.	1360 g.

NOTES

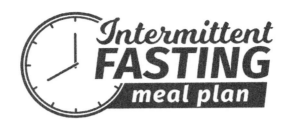

sunday

monday

tuesday

wednesday

thursday

friday

saturday

NOTES

Printed in Great Britain
by Amazon